THE MONTIGNAC METHOD
JUST FOR WOMEN

THE MONTIGNAC METHOD

...Just for Women

Michel Montignac

Montignac Publishing (UK) Ltd

First published in France under the title:
La Méthode Montignac...Spécial Femmes
1994

First published in UK 1995

ISBN 2 910907 00 7

www.montignac-publishing.com
info@montignac-publishing.com

TABLE OF CONTENTS

PART I

PREFACE

In this new book, which particularly emphasises women's needs, Michel Montignac again demonstrates that he not only has solid nutritional knowledge, but that he is also gifted with great insight into the subject.

There is no longer any doubt that he has achieved recognition as something of an expert in the nutritional field.

In the last few decades, medicine has made considerable progress, so that we can now better diagnose, treat and even prevent many diseases. Overall, our health has been greatly improved.

We have notably encouraged improvement in eating habits, as well as the practice of physical exercise. However, when we examine the problem of nutrition carefully, it has to be admitted that nothing worthwhile was really proposed before the advent of the Montignac method.

Whereas most dieticians were happy to lower weight and improve health with the simplistic method of reducing daily food intake, and particularly fats, Michel Montignac was the first to question the calorie theory approach and concentrate on the real relationship between various foods and the bio-chemical responses they provoke in the body.

Inspired by well-known studies which show why the French suffer less obesity and cardio-vascular illnesses than other industrialised nations and explain why, Michel Montignac

15

wisely postulated that the metabolic conversion of carbohydrates (and not that of fats and proteins) is the cornerstone of any nutritional programme.

Consumption of carbohydrates, leading to secretion of insulin, is the most important dietary factor.

If carbohydrates are chosen according to their glyceamic index, as recommended by Michel Montignac, secretion of insulin can be controlled, and as a consequence, weight gain or loss can be influenced.

The rules concerning consumption of fats and proteins, as defined by the Method, also lead to improvement in health. We know that proteins stimulate the secretion of glucagon, a hormone that indirectly contributes to a reduction in fat reserves.

Our services at the Mercy-Baptist Hospital in New-Orleans, U.S.A., have recently undertaken a study on the application of the principles of the Montignac Method.

The first results derived from study of our patients have shown not only a substantial reduction of excess fat, but also and above all, a lowering of between 20-30 % in their total cholesterol level in most cases.

We feel that these results are directly linked to the reduction in the secretion of insulin obtained with the Montignac Method. This is why we will now be undertaking in-depth studies in the course of which we will systematically measure insulin, cholesterol and triglycerides, and this should enable us to verify our hypotheses.

The Montignac Method represents an undoubted contribution to the nutritional field. It answers the questions that we ask concerning our eating habits in a scientific and rational manner. Before this Method, some things were unclear or had not been included.

If the Method is followed it can only lead to better health and greatly improved happiness.

I do not doubt that all serious studies undertaken in the

future will rapidly confirm that Michel Montignac was right to persevere in a new direction in which he will be recognised one day as a "pathfinder".

Doctor Morrison C. **BETHEA**
Head of Cardiac Surgery Department of the
Mercy-Baptist Hospital,
New-Orleans, U.S.A.

FOREWORD

Some people may wonder why is it necessary to publish a third book on the Montignac Method when the two previous books on the same subject have already achieved unprecedented sales.

Wouldn't it just be a "remake" and like Rambo II and III solely intended to artificially continue the successful sales of the first two books?

Were not *Dine out and lose weight* and *Eat yourself slim* enough to precisely reveal all the secrets of the Montignac Method? The number of readers' letters, as well as many press articles, and above all comments from some nutrition specialists proved to us that this was not the case.

The first book, written in 1986, was mostly for men, and particularly those eating out. The second one, *Eat yourself slim*, although giving an identical explanation of the basic principles of the Method, was more geared towards home eating and a feminine readership cooking most of their own meals.

The two works were essentially practical and intended to be simple in their approach. It was thought that an instructional, easily applied approach to learning about nutrition would have more substantial and long-lasting effects.

Behind the slimming method, however, was the outline of a precise nutritional theory leading to a really healthy

19

lifestyle. Readers would only realise this later when they felt the good physical effects of applying the recommendations that had led them to change their eating habits.

For self-evident practical reasons the original presentation was purposely simplified. What was the good of bombarding readers with an avalanche of scientific information that might only take their minds off the main issue?

This is why people had the idea for a long time that the Montignac Method was about separating (disassociating) starches and fats.

But, given our experience, it seemed that the disassociation message was far too simplistic even if it was good enough to get results. That is why from 1989/90 it was decided to include a chapter on glycaemic indexes upon which our nutritional principles are really based.

This additional explanation was not enough to stop malicious dieticians from continuing to present the Montignac Method as misconceived. Like for example the case of Doctor Jacques Fricker, who clumsily felt obliged to invent an "associative" diet to get media attention in relation to the Montignac Method. The latter can be resumed according to him by two principles inspired by Dr. Atkins: "the avoidance of carbohydrates and unbridled consumption of fats".

These erroneous allegations didn't fool anyone, certainly not general medical practitioners or cardio-vascular specialists, who have always noticed that when the Montignac Method is followed it leads to systematic regularisation of blood counts, notably for cholesterol and triglycerides in addition to substantial and lasting weight loss.

Publication of this third book is therefore justified for several reasons. Firstly, conclusions must be drawn from the teaching of a dietary approach that has largely proved itself in the last eight years, in view of how much it has been followed and the number of articles written about it.

It seems important and necessary now to repeat the essential teachings and to clarify or even redefine them.

If the Montignac Method has with time been accepted, this is because it is not a "diet" in the traditional restrictive and temporary sense of the term. Its success is more easily explained because, in addition to weight loss, it enables optimum vitality to be attained and above all can be seen to be a tool for better living and even fits into the concept of overall good health.

Most critical observers, particularly conventional nutritionists, have in fact misunderstood the real intentions of the first two books. They have deliberately only focused on the stringent rules of Phase I of the Method, over-emphasising its austerity and coming down too heavily on the exclusion of some foods.

Experience of practitioners in the field as well that from readers' letters has, on the contrary, shown us how much Phase I was only an intermediate stage which, although perfectly successful for those who followed it, and they stuck to it all the more because it is never restrictive, even if it is, and must be, selective. Everyone felt that after this transition period, the real principles of the Method would be found in Phase II, that is to say in a harmonious change in eating habits.

There were many readers however, who skimmed through Phase I and only remembered the main principles of the Method and stayed in the cruising phase. Their experience shows that they obtained the same results, but of course they needed more time to lose their pounds. This however, was more than beneficial on the level of weight stabilisation.

This is why we have chosen to present the Method in a different way. Henceforth, we will insist more on the fundamental principles, those which will lead us to understand how modern cultures have progressively adopted bad eating habits, the consequence of which is the dramatic increase in metabolic illnesses (overweight, diabetes and cardio-vascular disease in particular).

We will see how, by simple changes in our eating habits, making simple readjustments, the tendency can be completely reversed.

For women who have what might be termed an "addiction" to some foods (sugar for example), and for those who have a serious weight problem, or again, are in a hurry to see results, we will still propose Phase I (which can only be considered as an intermediate stage). They should thus be able to both radically change their bad habits by starting a real readjustment, give their body a rest so that it can find new health, and get very short term results. This "transitory" and "accelerated" phase will go back, more noticeably, to the place that it always had in the Method: that of an optional phase.

Thousands of the experiences that we have been able to gather from our readers over the years, have made us aware of the fact that application of the nutritional principles we recommend works differently according to sex.

Nevertheless, it is wrong to infer, as some have, that *"it works better for men than for women"*. We have always answered that we have seen the same benefits whichever the sex but that, for some women, it works differently.

There are several explanations to this phenomenon. Women who start out on the Method usually have a "very heavily loaded high calorie past". Some of them even have several decades of diets behind them The least that can be said is that their body is on the defensive and that any change in food, even a good one, necessarily comes up against a block.

A doctor from Rouen explained in this way the fact that one of his female patients had to wait seven months before she started to lose weight. The melting of her twenty-three extra pounds then occurred in a few weeks. She had been on restrictive diets for twenty-five years!

Besides its greater sensitivity, the female body is of greater complexity than that of her male counterpart. The hormonal implications are much more frequent and their secondary effects can in some cases favour weight gain, or at least slow down slimming. Women are, in addition, greater users of medicines. It turns out that some of these have contrary effects on the metabolism and can therefore indirectly act as a brake on slimming.

Merely changing the kind of medicine, without changing the necessary treatment, can be enough to unblock the situation.

For many years, doctors from the Institut Vitalité et Nutrition [1], as well as all those who have written to them, most of whom are working doctors, have contributed to a better understanding of the problem of weight gain as well as to that of resistance to weight loss, through their daily use of the Method with clients. It is therefore starting with their experience and with their help that it has been possible to write this book. Readers, and particularly women readers, will thus really be able to get maximum benefit from applying the principles of the Method and making it more effective.

---

1. Institut Vitalité et Nutrition: 1 rue Robin, 95880 Enghien-les-Bains, France. Tel: 00.33.1.39 83 18 39.

INTRODUCTION

In nature there is no such thing as being overweight, and even less being obese. There is virtually no trace of it in the animal kingdom, unless you look at domestic animals, and for good reason!

In primitive societies, obesity was generally very rare. These isolated cases could only be explained by a few serious health problems, notably of hormonal origin. In some tribes, it was this exceptional nature of obesity that gave rise to a veritable fatness cult. In fact, this *nec plus ultra* only occurred exceptionally.

In the following centuries, during the better documented great civilisations, obesity was generally the attribute of the rich, who because of their standard of living, had access to more "processed" food. Contrary to what you might first imagine, the wealthy in the past were fatter than the poor, not because they ate more, but because they ate differently. You will easily understand why from the following chapters.

Today, this tendency has been totally reversed as it is in the least favoured categories that we tend to find obesity, whilst amongst the richer people are slimmer.

To understand the current problem of obesity the best thing would be to go and study it in the country where it has become of such importance that it is a national catastrophe: the United States of America. There, 64 % of

Americans are too fat (as against 28 % in France), and 20 % are obese (as against 3 to 5 % in mainland France).

If History has shown us that obesity is a by-product of civilisation (as was the case in Egypt or the Roman Empire), it is understandable that this phenomenon is particularly visible today in the U.S.A. Doesn't this country effectively represent the most advanced model of modern civilisation, already well into its declining phase?

If you ask a specialised doctor why nature has given you "rather a lot of excess weight", having sworn by all the Gods that you eat nearly nothing and do a normal amount of physical exercise, he won't fail to trot out that old chestnut, the argument of heredity.

If a nutritionist or duty dietician can't manage to make you lose weight, don't expect them to question their dietary approach, as they will consider that it can only be your fault. If you really do not eat secretly, they think the only thing that can be responsible is your bad heredity.

It's true that as far as obesity is concerned heredity can give a strong predisposition, but it can't be blamed for everything. It is not necessarily, as it happens, "just fate" as you are often led to believe.

A hundred years ago, there was no obesity in the United States. By this I mean, not more than anywhere else. We cannot be expected to believe that since then the tens of millions of obese Americans in 1994 are descended from the few rare fat people who were the exception in the XIXth century, and that they have inherited their excess weight from their ancestors!

Strangely, most obese Americans are black today, whereas their African cousins from whom they are descended are not fat.

Something has happened then for the average weight of Americans to have progressively risen from generation to generation, especially as this phenomenon is recent as it only dates from the last few decades.

The idea cannot be dismissed that it is their bad eating habits that have progressively led them to develop the conditions for a bad heredity, which would show that the heredity factor is not innate but somehow acquired!

The second reason that is usually advanced by specialists to explain overweight and even more so obesity is "over-eating". In other words, that means to say that if people are fat it's because they eat too much.They will then insist that it is the rising standard of living and the consumer society that have made our contemporaries into inveterate "guzzlers" and immoral "gluttons"....when you think of the undernourished in the Third World!

If you look around you, you will be hard pressed to find the stereotype "fatty who eats all the time", caricatured so much in films.

You won't have a problem, on the other hand, digging out among your friends, acquaintances or even members or your own family, the model of the professional glutton, the one who is not only not fat but to cap it all is hopelessly thin.

They are the ones you will see always on the lookout for something that might finally make them put on a few pounds...

When you question fat people, you come to realise that except for a few, the amount of calories that they eat is incredibly low. Well, this paradox should not surprise us, as we will have the opportunity of showing later: the fatter people are, the more they despairingly count calories, and vice-versa.

If you were to find your grandparents' or even your parents' wedding, baptism and communion menus in your attic you would be amazed by the phenomenal quantity of food that they could ingurgitate at the time.

You will readily realise something that was proved long ago, that nowadays we eat somewhat poorly compared to them.

Then they will cleverly try to explain, with many details,

that if people could eat so much in the past it's because they used much more energy: they walked more often, took the trouble to walk up the stairs, lived in houses that were less well heated, etc.

This was probably true for some people, especially in the lower socio-professional classes, but if we analyse the situation of the middle classes of the time, you have to admit readily that they walked more for pleasure than out of necessity. Cars were perhaps less prevalent, but that did not mean that they ran around France with a bundle on their back like they did a few centuries ago.

Public transport and coaches were used much more than today. They certainly used the stairs more, but it must be said that there were far fewer stairs as tall buildings did not yet exist then.

As for central heating, it must be admitted that it was not as universal as it has become at the end of the 20th century and that, when it did exist, it was used sparingly. The throw away society had not yet emerged.

It is true though that people wore more clothes than today. The amount of clothes they wore was amazing, even in summer. The one fact largely compensates for the other.

Therefore, trying to make out that our contemporaries are fat because they eat too much energy in relation to the amount they use is not a convincing argument. That is why the explanation must be sought elsewhere.

It is quite clear that endemic obesity in Western societies can only be the result of the progressive change in our eating habits, those which we had practised for two centuries, and this has occurred above all since the last World War.

We will understand from the following chapter that obesity is not only directly linked to modern food fashions, but it is also the consequence of following successive low calorie diets.

But take heart, the explanations given in this book are very simple and the instructional method adopted will enable you to learn everthing about it.

The only thing that I would ask of you immediately is to make a small effort to read the few explanatory pages which you will find in the following chapters. Without this essential "preliminary" data it will be difficult for you to be able to put the nutritional principles of the Method into practice effectively.

I am always greatly saddened when I meet someone who says they have done, as they say wrongly, the "Montignac diet" and lost twenty pounds with no difficulty, and then regained half of it again afterwards.

It is always someone who has never "read" my book, but who has just been satisfied to use a few basic principles from it, out of context.

If these principles are applied without giving them some thought, they can effectively give rapid results, but once you have got to that point and followed them "to the letter" without having understood why you have lost weight, you will naturally be tempted to go back to your old eating habits.

The same causes lead to the same effects, and you will simply regain most of the lost pounds.

If you can recognise yourself in the picture that I have just painted, I would like to say again that the Montignac Method is not a "diet". It is a theory of living, leading to the adoption of new eating habits, essentially founded on good choices. When you have taken in the full details and the objectives, which is simple enough, applying these principles will be child's play.

If you have this book in your hands it is because you want to get rid of, once and for all, the extra pounds that are ruining your life.

By attentively reading the following chapters, you will first of all understand why traditional dietetics has lied to you in making you believe that all you had to do was to eat less to slim. You know no doubt by experience that this is not true.

In the second phase, you will understand why and how you have taken on the extra pounds. Finally, you will be convinced of the fact that there is only one serious solution to get rid of them for ever: EAT! but eat differently...

PART I

CHAPTER I

THE "STOVE" MYTH

It is clear from the previous explanation that obesity is a by-product of civilisation. But, even if throughout History the figures of some privileged people were a little stout – military leaders, aristocrats, the bourgeoisie or churchmen – it has to be recognised that obesity has always only been a marginal affliction.

It was not until the middle of the XXth century that the problem really became acute and took on the worrying proportions that we see now in the USA.

So it must be particular socio-cultural conditions which have presided over the blooming of this phenomenon. Fifty years or so ago in our societies food still had the significance that it had always had for centuries: "the life source".

Everyone was convinced of the way in which food influenced their health and that their food was "their best medicine", as Hippocrates stated five centuries before Christ.

Food had even more importance at the time as it was scarce and expensive. Even a few decades ago, in fact, the spectre of famine, or at least of shortages, even restrictions, was still present in everyone's mind.

Today's shopping basket has become the consumer trolley and is overloaded with abundance. Food has become so obtainable that the wastage that most of us indulge in has become an insult to the starving of the Third World.

Henceforth we no longer earn our bread by the sweat of our brow, for the dustbins are full of it. In the past household leftovers were carefully re-used or else regularly collected to feed animals. Nowadays, they go straight off to join the rest of the rubbish that the consumer society produces!

It needed an important event for this disrespectful attitude to gradually develop over food. This event can only be called the "food plethora". It is this which came out of the agro-food revolution at the end of the Second World War and made our daily "manna" banal, changing the ways people thought.

Since 1945 our society has had to face two major problems:
(1) a big increase in population, following the post-war baby boom and the advent of tens of thousands of refugees;
(2) intensive urbanisation as a consequence of the latter phenomenon, but also the progressive depopulation of the countryside

Therefore more had to be produced, and produced differently, as for the first time in the history of humanity there was a sudden discrepancy between the food production zones and the consumption zones.

In 1950, 80 % of what was consumed in a provincial town was produced in the 50 kilometres around it. The other 20 % came from neighbouring areas or further afield. Today the ratio is completely reversed. In addition, when food was produced on the spot the waste and leftovers were recycled as fertiliser.

When food was transported away from the production area nothing could be recuperated and it became necessary to resort to other fertilisation methods.

In the last fifty years the agricultural industry has continually developed, relying on a large spread of technologies, each more productive than the last. This revolution has had several consequences:

1. Productivity could be considerably increased by:

1.1. mechanisation;
1.2. massive use of chemical fertilisers;
1.3. generalisation of use of pesticide, insecticides and fungicides;
1.4. the organisation of intensive industrial scale breeding.

2. Preservation techniques could be developed through:

2.1. generalisation of refrigeration and freezing;
2.2. the use of food additives and other chemical preservatives.

The result of all these measures was in fact far greater than predicted, which means that a whole sector of humanity was able to enter into a phase of food abundance.

From the beginning of this period of transformation of the agricultural industry picture, observers did not fail to see that the average weight of the Western population rose in a very significant way.

In the United States, from the 1930's, they began to seek solutions to the problem of obesity. The scientists of the time (dietetics and nutrition were not considered as medical specialities then) pondered the question and developed a hypothesis: if the average weight of the population was suddenly rising, at a time when the West was entering a veritable era of food over-abundance, it was likely that there was a relationship of cause and effect. This is how the "stove" myth was born.

They thought that the human body works like a stove. To survive, it needs energy provided by its food. On the one hand then there were the energy inputs, and on the other the expenditure.

Plumpness, and even more so, obesity, could therefore only be the consequence of an imbalance between the "receipts" and the "debits". In other words, the extra pounds were only residual energy.

So, there were only two solutions, either there was too high an input, or the expenditure of energy was not high enough.

That therefore meant that if you were fat, it was either because you ate too much or you did not do enough exercise, or both together.

From this simplistic hypothesis, which nevertheless followed a certain logic, the theory of calorie excess was elaborated. Since energy inputs could be measured in calorie unit values, all foods could thus be classified according to their calorie power, weight and the category to which they belonged (carbohydrates, fats, proteins).

However, this reasoning was already flawed at birth, as calories were only counted on the plate without taking into consideration what really happened during the digestive process.

It was from this that conventional dietetics was born. It was intentionally restrictive as it was of a calorie theory nature. By deciding that the human body needed about 2 500 calories a day, it also explained that depending on your real energy consumption you could change your weight in either direction.

Thus, if you consumed 3 000 calories a day you would have an excess of 500 calories, which would be stored, leading to a weight increase.

If, on the other hand, you stuck to 2 000 calories you would then be short of 500 calories, and the body would be forced to dig into its reserves to compensate for the difference which would then lead to loss of weight.

In other words, the calorie theory applied to nutrition postulated that to slim you only had to eat less and consequently if you got fatter it was because you ate too much.

It was this simplistic schematic theory, founded on a naive belief, which prevailed in dietetics in the last few decades. Well, it is unfortunately the one that is officially still put forward in hospital nutrition units and the one that is taught still in dietetic schools.

Reasoning according to the energy model, as all the professionals in dietetics still do, leads to a deliberate disregard for the phenomena of adaptation and regulation of the human body. This is to deny personal differences which make each individual unique, and in addition pass over the influence of the quality factor for food.

Contrary to what is generally accepted, an obese person is not necessarily someone who eats too much. In most cases, it is even the reverse. Statistics obtained from obese populations (in France as well as all the other Western countries), show that:

- Only 15 % of obese people eat too much (2 800 to 4 000 calories);
- 35 % of fat people eat normally (2 000 to 2 700 calories);
- 50 % of fat people eat little (800 to 1 500 calories).

¨n the world of competitive sport it can even be seen that to maintain a stable weight, the amount of calories can vary from 2 500 to 9 000, not because of the kind of sport but according to the individual.

Alain Mimoun, the marathon runner, maintained his weight and kept up his rigorous training on only 2 000 calories a day, whilst the competitive cyclist Jacques Anquetil needed 6 000 calories to keep his weight level and remain fit.

Even though medical literature remains curiously silent on this subject a good many studies have, however, been published which show that the difference in calorie intake is insignificant whether the subjects are thin, normal, fat or obese. In reality, there is no significant correlation between size and the energy intake.

But, the best way of being convinced of the ineffectiveness

of the calorie theory approach is to analyse the results in the country where it is daily present: the United States.

Ninety million Americans have constantly followed low calorie diets in the last forty-five years. The calorie message is all pervasive there. Through audio-visual communications and especially advertising, this dietetic culture has been permanently rooted in their minds.

And to be certain of getting results, Americans, who always go overboard, do not only count calories, but also more or less obsessionally throw themselves into physical exercise to be sure to burn up the maximum of energy.

Well now, statistics concerning obesity in the United States show us a catastrophic situation.

Whilst more than one third of the population religiously follows low calorie diets and does daily intense physical exercise, paradoxically the Americans are the fattest people in the world.

Two thirds of the population is excessively fat, as against one third in France, and one American in five is obese as against one in twenty in France. All this, even though it is not really possible to compare the relatively obese French to the super-obese Americans, for it is frequent to meet people in America who weigh over 660 pounds (more than 41 stone).

A documentary made on obesity in the USA which was shown in November 1990 on the French television channel TF1, showed a specimen who reached 1014 pounds (over 63 stone), and the Guinness Book of Records, for its part gives the heaviest weight ever achieved by a human being as 1368.852 pounds (nearly eighty-five and a half stone). It was, of course, someone of American citizenship.

It is true that if we really want to understand why the low calorie diets which have been proposed for the last forty years are doomed to failure, the easiest place to verify it is in the USA.

But, in all the Western countries where they have been

applied with a degree of perseverance, the results are similar, that is to say, a catastrophe.

We knew that low calorie diets were ineffective, since their application always leads to failure. Now we know why. The hypothesis they are based upon is false and has no scientific basis. We will see even, in the following chapters, that they are dangerous.

CHAPTER II

RED HERRINGS OR
"THE BAD SLIMMING GUIDE"

Low calorie diets: danger!

We saw previously how the concept of the energy balance for the human body was developed historically, together with the idea of low calorie diets which are its practical application. We can stand back far enough now to be able to see its ineffectiveness.

Professor David Gartner from the University of Michigan considers, together with many of his colleagues, that the first determining factor of obesity in the USA is the *"following of successive low calorie diets"*. It is then really low calorie diets which lead to a "dietetic of failure". But, even if everyone can see it, to be convinced this must be demonstrated.

All those, especially women, who have at some time followed a low calorie diet know that, at first, you generally get results, but you never manage to keep stable.

Worse still, in many cases, you can even find yourself subsequently with a further weight gain. We are going to try to understand why by examining the body's behaviour.

Let us imagine that the daily ration for an individual is around 2 500 calories and that she has been bothered by a few extra pounds. If we lower this calorie ration to 2 000 calories, as in the classical low calorie theory approach, we will have created a deficit of 500 calories

The organism, which is used to receiving 2 500 calories, will therefore feel deprived and will take the equivalent of the 500 missing calories from the reserve fats. You will therefore get a corresponding weight loss.

After a time, which will vary from one individual to another, it will be noticed that slimming no longer occurs even though the low calorie diet has been adhered to. This is because there will be a progressive adjustment between the "credits" and "debits".

As the body is now only getting 2 000 calories a day, it decides to manage with that and you see weight stagnating.

If you are intent on going on with the experiment because you think that the weight loss may continue after you have got past the levelling off point, disappointment will be even greater. You will in fact find that the weight curve will take off steadily in an upwards direction.

Paradoxically, while you are eating less you are putting on weight again. The explanation is simple. The human body is in fact moved by the survival instinct which begins to act as soon as it is menaced by a restriction of intake. As the reduction in energy input has continued for some time, the body, after having adjusted its outgoings to match the incoming energy, is led by its survival instinct to further reduce its expenditure. This may go down to 1 700 calories, for example, to enable the reserves to build up again.

It must not be forgotten that shortages, due to droughts and other causes of famine in the old days are not such far removed events, and that though the memory remains in the subconscious, it can resurface at the least signal.

In fact, the human body still has the same survival instinct as a dog that buries its bones even though it is dying of hunger. Oddly, it is always when it is starving that an animal calls upon its sense of self-preservation to build up reserves.

In addition, when the body is in a situation of need, that is to say, undernourished, it is particularly on the defensive and misses no opportunity to build reserves when the occasion arises.

Those who are used to low calories diets also know very well that the least deviation from the diet, during a weekend for example, can make them regain, all in one go, the five to seven pounds that they have taken weeks to lose.

This is also one of the reasons why we advise our readers never to miss a meal, as many people nevertheless do. If you deny yourself food for one meal, the body panics, and because of the frustration it has been subjected to, takes advantage of the next meal to build reserves.

The habit of only feeding the dog once a day (for evident practical reasons) is just as silly and can in many cases explain a pet's weight problem.

The experiments which have been done on laboratory animals have also shown quite clearly that for the same quantity of daily food, animals that only had one meal, in the long term became obese and those that received the equivalent of five or six meals spread over the day kept to an optimum weight.

We have already noted that female obesity could be more difficult to combat than that of males, and this is linked to the special physiology of women. We will speak of this problem in detail in the second part of this book.

In Part II of this book, we notably give the reasons why there is more fatty tissue in the female body than in that of the male – this is because the number of fat cells is greater.

We have known for a long time that obesity in women (and in men) leads to an increase in the volume of each fat cell, but it also leads to (and it is this that gives it its specificity) multiplication in the number of these cells. The drama is even greater as this situation cannot be reversed.

Although it is possible to succeed in lowering the volume

of a fat cell, it is impossible to reduce their number when it has increased.

Additionally, studies have shown that it is above all in cases where the intake of food is restricted (low calorie diet) that the female body calls upon its survival instinct and manufactures new fat cells. It is unfortunately this procedure that enables it, subsequently, to recover its lost fat even more quickly, and above all increase its volume, its potential having thereby become greater.

A low calorie diet is not only illusory and ineffective, as we have shown, it is additionally dangerous, as it will have the effect of consolidating the female propensity to obesity by an insidious increase in the capital of fat cells in the long term.

When we study the background of an obese person (more than thirty to forty pounds above a normal weight), we see that in most cases the greater part of this overweight has been built up over several years, by going on successive low calorie diets.

It is easy to see from the above example how, with a starting weight which was stable at ninety kilos, and a food intake of 3 000 calories, an individual can find himself a few years later at two hundred and sixty four pounds (120 kilos), even though he is only eating 800 calories.

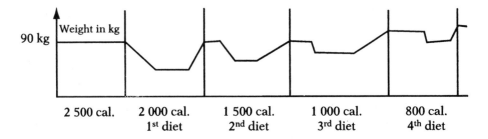

90 kg	Weight in kg				
	2 500 cal.	2 000 cal. 1st diet	1 500 cal. 2nd diet	1 000 cal. 3rd diet	800 cal. 4th diet

Tribulations of the under-nourished or the martyrdom of the obese

44

It can be seen that each time that a low calorie diet was started, there followed three stages: slimming, stabilisation and recovery of weight. What it is important to note is that when new diets are undertaken, they are less and less productive.

In the beginning the weight curve goes back more or less to the starting level then, gradually as it goes on in time and increased weight gain occurs.

This is why because they obstinately wanted to lose ten pounds, when they had become stable at a certain level, some people find themselves fifteen years later with a weight gain of sixty pounds, while at the same time they are completely undernourished.

Every day doctors tell us that they have met amongst their clients patients who at the price of severely controlled rationing and enormous frustrations (brought about by the 800 calorie diets) still not only cannot slim, but most often continue to put on weight.

The situation is even more dramatic as with such "poverty diets", these people are completely lacking in indispensable nutrients (essential fatty acids, mineral salts, vitamins, oligo-elements), which makes them feel very tired and also much more vulnerable to illness, as their defence mechanisms have been reduced.

In addition, many of them find that they become completely depressed or even anorexic or bulimic.

They then only have to change specialist; quit the dietician to land up at the psychiatrists.

Finally, these "see-saw obesities" make the appearance of cardio-vascular illnesses more likely, even in the absence of high cholesterol, diabetes or smoking.

Professor Bronwell of the University of Pennsylvania studied the phenomenon in laboratory rats who were fed alternately rich and poor calorie diets.

The animals gained and lost weight, but the rhythm of gain and loss varied for each new diet. During the first diet, the rat lost weight in twenty-one days and regained it

45

in forty-six days. During the second diet, the rat lost the same weight in fifty-six days and regained it all in fourteen days. From then on the weight loss was obtained with more and more difficulty and the gain was quicker and faster. Thus it was proved that the metabolism can adapt itself to a calorie reduction.

Any calorie deficit can in fact reduce the metabolic expenditure of the body by more than 50 % but, on the other hand, any return to normal, even for a short period, is accompanied by a sudden regain of weight. Finally, the greater the gap between the diet and normal food intake, the more rapidly weight gain will happen,

The effect of these "see-saw diets" that lead to a yo-yo like variation of weight and to a progressive resistance to any slimming is well known, but paradoxically it is only quietly decried by specialists, as though there were a kind of conspiracy of silence. It would be a bit like being afraid today of admitting that for forty-five years one has been completely wrong.

However, the recent initiative of Professor Apfelbaum must be acknowledged. During the International Conference in Anvers in September 1993, he gave a positive answer to his own question: *"As far as treatment of obesity is concerned, have we not been collectively wrong?"*

Funnily enough, the public itself, which is nevertheless the first to pay the cost and suffer, is not always ready to accept the truth.

One day I took advantage of the invitation I had received to take part in a big television debate on obesity to try, without much success, to speak for a few minutes on the subject. The broadcast was pre-recorded and that part was simply cut from the broadcast version, most probably because no-one was interested!

A journalist, well known for her serious articles on health, tells the story of how she once published a long article denouncing low calorie diets and explaining, as we have just done, their dangers. Result: absolutely nothing. Not one letter from readers. Total indifference, whilst the many "miracle diets" are always extremely successful.

It must be said the "low calorie phenomenon" has, in our Western societies, acquired a truly cultural dimension. It has even been, here as elsewhere, and notably on the American continent, institutionalised at every level.

How can a principle that still remains intact in the programmes of all the medical faculties, and even forms the basis of the teaching given in the official dietetic schools, is used by all collective restaurants in hospitals, schools and businesses be questioned?

How can you question a principle that is an important undercurrent in the economic structure of our Western societies?

The agricultural industry (food farming) is more than successful today. It is even in some countries, like France, the leading industry and one of the most prosperous.

When you go to an exhibition such as the SIAL [1] you realise that all the objectives of these businesses in terms of their development, are conceived with the low calorie theory in mind.

All the marketing studies are formal: this is the direction in which to move, this is the market of tomorrow! All the new products that are coming out will therefore be formulated with this in mind. However, the "light" foods have lost ground over the years.

Hotel chains have also caught the low calorie virus. Many of them already have low calorie meals on their menus in their restaurants. Others have separate sections where, instead of a Maître d'Hôtel a dietician is in charge.

---

1. SIAL: a large international exhibition for the food industry which is held every November in Villepinte, near the Charles de Gaule airport outside Paris.

"Deceptive" protein packages

Amongst the lowest low calorie approaches must be noted the VLCD diets (very low calorie diet) which are based on proteins in package form.

This protein diet, which should theoretically be reserved for serious obesity (those with a BMI above 30 [2]) is unfortunately still prescribed by some practising doctors and is even among the medications that women prescribe for themselves without any proper medical supervision.

1. What is the principle?

They are based on substituting 55 to 75 grams of protein powder (to be diluted) or a pre-prepared liquid for normal food for twenty to thirty days. These proteins give about 500 calories a day (and sometimes less).

They are complemented by vitamin and mineral supplements as well as plenty to drink (at least two litres a day).

The protein content of these packages prevents muscular wasting and the fact that they contain no carbohydrates reduces blood glucose level (glycaemia) and insulin secretion. The latter also enables acetone compounds to be produced which cut the appetite within 48 hours and give the subject a feeling of slight euphoria.

The body is then forced to make glucose using reserve fat: new blood sugar is then produced. When these fat reserves melt, this is called lipolisis and the subject loses weight.

2. What are their defects?

Scientific studies undertaken on different parts of the body have shown that there is muscle (protein) wastage during

---

2. Body Mass Index: See Chapter I, Part II.

the first nineteen days and that their level only balances out from the twentieth day.

Nearly 25 % of the weight loss is caused in the non-fatty muscular tissue. But, it is true that in obesity, the non-fatty tissue also increases.

A high level of salt loss in addition also leads to loss of water which always has an effect on the scales, and care must be taken to see that this does not lead to possible fall in blood pressure.

This lowering of blood pressure is due to the absence of starches, which leads to a loss of sodium and water.

When the diet stops, starches must be reintroduced very slowly, as if they are absorbed in large quantities, they will cause oedemas because of sudden water retention.

The secondary effects of VLCD are many:
- an increase in the level or uric acid: 10 to 20 %;
- a fall in blood pressure: from 8 to 10 %;
- hair loss: 9 %
- constipation: 8 to 10 %
- tiredness: 8 %
- broken nails: 8 %
- dry skin: 8 %
- intolerance to cold: 8 %
- muscular cramps: 7 %
- menstruation difficulties: 6 %
- depression: 5 %
- headaches: 3 %

Hyperuricemia (a high level of uric acid) continues for about three weeks. To limit the risks (gout attacks or the appearance of nephratis because of the formation of stones in the bladder) it is essential to drink lots of water.

Constipation is normal as there is no input of solid foods. It can be countered by eating salads seasoned with lemon juice.

The most dramatic complication which can very occasionally occur is sudden death. The food and Drug Admin-

49

istration counted seventeen deaths due to these "very low calorie diets" in the USA!

These were, as it happens, women who with no previous record had succumbed to heart attacks and an irreversible cardiac arrest. In thirteen cases, the proteins taken were of bad quality. They were poor in tryptophane and the necessary potassium supplement had been omitted.
In the four other cases, no evident cause was found, but for being on the treatment for five or six months, whereas protein diets must not be used for more than four weeks.

When we know that these "treatments" are freely on sale in chemists, we can only be horrified, as they should be prescribed only to patients who have a body mass index above thirty [3], and having previously had a complete check-up for their kidney and cardiac functions. The diet should not be started again for at least three months.
It follows that these diets must be undertaken under the control of a competent medical team, in a hospital environment, and with strict cardiac surveillance.
However, how can it be ensured that once they have been intoxicated by the promising results obese people are not tempted to continue the treatment for more than two months?

For women who only occasionally follow this kind of diet for eight to ten days they should be aware that for the first week they provoke muscular wasting and loss of water. There is no decrease in fat tissue and that is why they do not lose weight!
These draconian deprivations do not even guarantee them sure weight loss since, as the study made by Van Goal has shown, out of four hundred cases, there were only:

– 38 % success over six months;
– 31 % over a year:
– 14 % over two years.

---

3. See Chapter I, Part II.

50

With hindsight, a recent study published by the University of Pennsylvania even indicated only a 2 % success rate over five years.

Professor Apfelbaum, who was even an ardent supporter of this protein diet for more than twenty-five years, had the courage, at the International Conference on Obesity in Anvers in 1993, to recognise its uselessness, concluding that *in the long term, all the patients regained their lost kilos*.

The worst thing is that in spite of the dangers (when they are used without surveillance), these treatments are even more readily available as they constitute a lucrative market for pharmaceutical companies and chemists. When they are bought directly (through mail order) on a Doctor's prescription, the latter still receives a percentage on the volume sold, which goes to prove that any profit is a good profit!

Such an approach to slimming is basically flawed as it creates an artificial four week "holiday" period in the "food life" of the patient, who thereby bypasses the real problems. The patient (usually a woman) then has no sense of a long-term framework for a slimming project directed towards the modification of food habits, which would need the patient to be supported and supervised.

It is only by shopping at the grocer's, the market or supermarket, but certainly not at the chemists, that a serious nutritional step can be made on the path to weight loss.

"Irritating" meal substitutes

Nowadays, the windows and shelves of chemists have been invaded by vanilla and chocolate flavoured packets of powders which, taken at breakfast or lunch, are supposed to make you slimmer. In the evening you have the honour of being able to eat a "normal" dinner.

Their chemical composition varies greatly, but is always

unbalanced. Some of them are lacking in proteins and others contain too many sugary carbohydrates.

Let us see why this option is even more perverse.

Amongst the mechanisms that calm hunger pangs, on the one hand can be grouped chewing, and on the other the feeling of satisfaction (full stomach).

If you swallow a liquid, however, you neither chew nor feel that you have eaten enough, and this is quite simply because "it doesn't stay in the body". Result: a few hours later you are hungry and the risk of snacking is even greater.

If these substitutes have been taken in the morning and at lunch time (at the times when "getting fatter" is less likely), you will be tempted to eat a very substantial dinner. Bad luck! This just the time when the body is more inclined to build reserves, and even more so because it will have been frustrated by the two previous pseudo-meals. This brings us back to the calorie theory again!

In addition, there is an obvious psychological mistake in opting for meal substitutes as fat women who do so, or even those who are just a bit overweight, will unconsciously develop a kind of aversion to food which they will gradually come to think of as being responsible for all their troubles.

They will then reinforce their feeling that food is the enemy and has to be regarded with caution whilst we think the opposite message must be given. Obese women must first of all come to terms with their food instead of rejecting it wholesale. They will then learn to make the right choices.

Miracle medicines

The "miracle pill" that will make you thin, is still one of our dreams. But, to be acceptable on the medical and ethical level it has to meet a certain number of criteria:

– effectiveness proved by reliable and repeatable experiments;
– it is well supported (absence of undesirable side-effects);
– absence of toxicity in the long term.

Evidently then, this pill, which looks very like a blue moon, is not for tomorrow, as for the moment no product comes anywhere near to matching this ideal model!
We can however study remedies offering a hope of slimming which have been prescribed in the past or which are, unfortunately, still on the market.

1. Diuretics

If "slimming" means losing a certain amount of fatty tissue, it is obvious that diuretics, which only cause water loss by forcing the body to urinate abundantly, do not in any way meet this objective.
In addition, it must be noted that water takes with it mineral salts (sodium, potassium), and this eventually leads to more bad than good: dry skin, tiredness, muscular cramps and giddiness, to which can be added lowering of blood pressure which can lead to fainting. When the treatment stops, the body has, in addition, a tendency to react like a sponge which has been under pressure for a long time: it regains its water more quickly, together with its salt, and as a bonus runs the risk of appearance of oedemas which can be hard to get rid of.
Doctors who still have the cheek to prescribe diuretics (which are as useless as they are dangerous) only rarely are honest enough to write the names out in full as they are easily recognised and usually prescribed for the treatment of well-known diseases. This is why they often hide them by using chemical terms which are unknown to their patients, or by quietly incorporating them into generic pseudo-homeopathic preparations.

In the same category, some plant remedies which are prescribed should be viewed with caution when they recommend the use of "drainers" which, while seemingly natural, contain plants with a more or less obvious diuretic effect.

Amongst these we can name horsetail, fennel, burdock, meadow sweet, artichoke, dandelion, ash, cherry stalks, etc.

Their diuretic effects may be slight, which reduces the risks of potassium loss, but they still cause water loss.

As for mineral water, which is often presented as an aid to slimming, generally its only grace is as a marketing ploy. Of course you must drink enough, but as we have already stated, it can only have slightly diuretic effects. Even if drinking does effectively help to get rid of waste from protein metabolism (urine, uric acid), it is not likely to get rid of fat!

2. Laxatives

Some women cleverly think that they can slim by simply passing faeces!

They will learn that they mainly risk damaging their colon by using irritating laxatives, or creating potassium deficiencies because of the diarrhoea which results from the stupid use of "cleansers". These women are only showing a phobic (fear of "poisons") or obsessional (constantly worrying about cleanliness) tendency.

3. Thyroid extracts

Thyroid deficiency is only occasionally a cause of obesity. Prescribing thyroid extracts to a patient whose thyroid is working properly is not only useless, but dangerous, as it can lead to a false hyper-thyroid condition.

These medicines which reduce muscle rather than fat, also run the risk of causing cardiac rhythm disturbance as the heart, it must be remembered, is also a muscle (though of course a rather different one).

Because of the secondary effects they engender (by unbalancing the thyroid), these thyroid extracts often have bad side effects. Difficulties occur which combine insomnia, anxiety, palpitations, tachycardia, irregular heartbeat, trembling and nervousness.

However, the worst complication remains sudden fall in blood pressure in an already existing heart condition (angina) which may not have been noticed in a previous check.

There again, these poison-remedies are often hidden in complex compounds and masked by the use of complicated chemical names or of cryptic abbreviations. Plant therapies often prescribe various algae and vesicle fucus which act on the thyroid through the intermediary of their iodine content.

4. Appetite depressants

These are compounds of amphetamines which cut the appetite as well as having a psychologically stimulating effect. It is no surprise to find then that they lead to a state of excitement which causes sleeping difficulties as well as lowering of self-esteem and self-control.

Though their greatest drawback remains that when they are stopped they frequently lead to nervous depression which can go as far as suicide, their greatest defect is that they can cause a bad case of dependency which can lead on to addiction.

It is easy to become a real appetite depressor junkie!

The obese person who eats often and little is spared this, but for those (particularly women) who suffer from eating disturbances (bulimia), taking amphetamines can only aggravate the problem.

5. Adifax

Pharmaceutical companies have tried to develop a molecule which while keeping certain beneficial effects of amphetamines would be les risky and without further bad side effects.

This is how dexfenfluramin came into being, which is better known under the name of Adifax, and which has overcome the psychological stimulation effect. According to the experiments that have taken place on animals, it would not lead to dependency.

It works by modifying the metabolism of serotonin, a substance which is implicated in appetite control and leads to a feeling of satisfaction. Its efficiency was seen on patients who had compulsive carbohydrate behaviour, in other words, sugar fanatics, but the latter in fact only account for 15 % of obesity.

A double blind study, with a placebo [4] control group, was carried out on more than eight hundred obese people for a year. Eighty-six per cent of the women were more than 40 % over the average weight in relation to the ideal weight theory (with a BMI on average of 32). This study proved that the treatment had side effects.

It must be noted that these people were also following a low calorie diet of less than 1 450 calories a day, and that they were supervised and counselled. Nearly 40 % of the patients had to stop the treatment because of bad side effects: tiredness, upset stomach, headaches, sleep difficulties, diarrhoea, dry mouth, anxiety, depression, frequent urination, feeling faint, drowsiness, sickness and vomiting.

In the eleventh month the difference in weight between the group treated with dexfenfluramin and the one treated with the placebo was only about 2.7 kilograms on an average.

---

4. Placebo: a neutral substance which is used in the place of a medicine.

Going over the results two months after the treatment was stopped (it lasted a year), it was noted that the placebo group of patients had regained one kilo per month, and those taking Adifax had regained two!

The doctors who did this study concluded therefore that the treatment had to be lifelong to maintain its very relative effectiveness (which greatly pleased the pharmaceutical company).

What we see here leads us to ask a certain number of questions:

- is it really necessary and above all reasonable to take two Adifax pills a day for a year to lose 2.7 kilos more than would be lost with a placebo?
- is the excessive cost of this treatment, which is not normally covered by the National Health Service justified for such small results?
- What would have been the effect of the medicine if taken alone (without the low-calorie diet)?
- In the final analysis, what share could be attributed to the low-calorie diet and what to the psychological support therapy?
- Would patients rather risk a slow weight gain after a year by continuing the therapy or a speedy one by stopping it?

In addition, as we mentioned above, if of the 15 % of people concerned there were one third who gave up, there were only really 10 % of the obese who achieved some relative benefit from this treatment with the slim hope of being able to lose three kilos (under seven pounds) more than with a classic treatment.

Knowing that the cost of this treatment was a "pipe dream" of around £70 odd per two pounds of fat lost, it is only right to ask if it was worth the risk! The gain seems, in any case, rather little (at least for the patient!).

The therapeutic answer to an eating disorder cannot and must not be reduced to prescribing a medicine, without the necessary psychotherapy (or behaviour therapy) which should be part re-educating food habits. Even if many of the women who are impatient to slim to get into their bathing costume from time to time when the holidays are coming up, hope to be able to fall back on a miracle drug, doctors should have reservations about it. Prescriptions should not be written out hurriedly for the short term. This is all the more true as some medicines (as well as being toxic and having side effects) expose their users to serious medical complications: the rebound of the therapy when weight is regained.

Constant recourse to these inconsistent therapies will lead to resistance to slimming with, contrary to the intended aim, constant rise in obesity.

Once again, any slimming strategy can only be conceived in a long-term perspective, being aware of current food fads. The decision to slim must be a maturely thought out choice, and that is why spectacular instant solutions will only lead to future disappointments.

A second look at food supplements

If you are into lightning solutions, watch out for the many slimming aid products that are sold with misleadingly natural-sounding names.

1. L-Carnitine

L-Carnatine is an enzyme which is found in the organism. It is synthesised in the liver and kidneys from two amino-acids: L-Lysin and L-Methionin, with the help of iron and vitamins C and B6.

Nowadays, L-Carnitine deficiency is in fact very rare, as we can obtain this enzyme from foods that we eat regularly: meat, chicken, rabbit, cow's milk and eggs.

Only a few vegetarians, notably women who have little iron in their diet, possibly might not synthesise L-Carnitine properly.

There are some extremely rare congenital deficiencies in L-Carnitine and people who suffer from these may have muscular troubles but they are not obese!

L-Carnitine is wrongly advertised as a substance which will help to "burn up fat". Let us look into this claim. It is certainly necessary for the use of free fatty acids in the blood but as "an energy fuel", but in no way does it burn fat reserves which are stored as triglycerides

Only when another enzyme is activated, triglyceride-lipasis (when the insulin level is low) can it help to melt reserve fats and free fatty acids into the blood stream.

Luckily, the Fraud Squad in France has forbidden the sale of many of the products containing L-Carnitine. In the near future it should only be a bad memory. No doubt other miracle products will take its place!

2. Plants

Plant therapies (phytotherapy) have now been called to the rescue: fat-eating plants, diuretic teas, fucus patches, any carrot for those who want to slim without making an effort and who will eat anything to do so!

Take the example of pineapple. Who has not heard tell at least once in their life that pineapple melts fat? The well-known bromelin or bromelaine which is in fact found in the stalk and not in the fruit itself by no means lives up to its reputation as a "fat eater" for slimming. It does not even have the beneficial effects on the metabolism of insulin that it was thought to. As for bean pods, they have gone slightly out of fashion since they caused intestinal blockages in the United States.

Other plants that were thought to be inoffensive have also turned out to be toxic and have now been taken off the market.

The same goes for some of the Chinese slimming plants (the more exotic the more people like it) which have been responsible for very serious toxic hepatitis. The only substances that can, possibly, be defended are soluble fibres like glucomane, but they have no effect in small doses.

At 4 grams a day they can work to cut down cravings. If they are taken with a large glass of water, half an hour before a meal they blow up the stomach, give a feeling of already being full up and lower the amount of insulin secreted. But they also tend to create uncomfortable wind in the stomach.

Whatever they do or whatever pill they succumb to it will inevitably take the mind of a fat person off the real aim: long-lasting modification of their eating habits. It is only when this nutritional objective has been fully understood that weight can be stabilised in the long term.

CHAPTER III

NUTRITIONAL COMPOSITION OF FOODS

It has become clear from the preceding chapters that it is not the energy contained in foods that is responsible for weight gain.

Subsequently, we will see that what makes all the difference is the nature of the food, that is to say, its nutritional content in terms of glucides (carbohydrates), lipids (fats) and proteins, fibres, vitamins, mineral salts and oligo-elements (trace elements).

We will then see then that fatness does not occur because of over-eating, but because of bad eating habits and because good food choices are not always made.

We can resume this by saying that to lose weight and find your ideal weight, depriving yourself of food serves no purpose. We will soon understand that it is enough to eat more harmoniously by avoiding some bad foods and eating more beneficial ones instead.

But to make good choices, you first of all have to be able to see clearly amongst the various categories of foods that are available and understand each of their characteristics.

This chapter, in spite of its technical nature, will be easily understood by all women readers, even if they do not have much of a scientific background.

Whatever your second fiddle or your hobby may be (i.e. gardening, DIY, sports), or whatever your profession (office worker, etc.), the first thing that you learn when you start are the "basic principles". From these you can then begin to make serious progress.

Some of the information that you will be given herein will seem familiar to you, but read carefully as so many false things have been said about the nutrition field that it is best to be careful.

The first thing you need to know is that all foods are made up of nutrients, that is to say substances which can be assimilated by the body and are intended to support life.

These nutrients can be grouped into two categories:

Energy providing nutrients

Their role is to not only provide energy but also to serve as raw materials for many of the processes of synthesis that go into the construction and the reconstruction of living matter. They include:

- proteins
- glucides or carbohydrates;
- lipids or fats.

Non-energy providing nutrients

- fibres;
- water;
- mineral salts;
- oligo-elements;
- vitamins.

Energy Providing Nutrients

1. Proteins

The proteins are organic substances, of animal or vegetable origin, which form the support for the cell structures of the body. They are made up of numerous amino acids which are their basic elements.

Whilst some of these amino acids can be manufactured by the body, others, can only be supplied by food, as the body does not know how to synthesise them itself.

Proteins can have two sources:

- *animal*: they can be found in meat, offal, and pork products (ham, sausages, etc.), fish, crustaceans (lobster, shrimp, etc.) shellfish, eggs, and milk products including cheese;
- *vegetable*: they can be found in soya, seaweed, almonds, hazelnuts, chocolate, and also in cereals, whole foods and pulses.

A sufficient supply of protein is indispensable for:

- the building of cell structures;
- manufacture of some hormones and neuro-transmitters such as thyroxin and adrenaline;
- as a possible source of energy for the organism if needed;
- to maintain the muscle system;
- for the formation of bile acids and respiratory pigments.

Cordon-bleu cooks please note! No food, apart from the egg, gives us such a complete and well balanced cocktail of amino acids. When you realise that the absence of an indispensable amino acid can be a "limiting factor" and can hinder assimilation of the others, you will understand even better why it is particularly recommended that your food should come from both animal and vegetable sources.

Meals which are made up only of vegetables, such as some

63

people concoct, necessarily lead to an imbalance, whereas a vegetarian diet which includes eggs and milk products is entirely acceptable (see Chapter IV, Part II).

However, if protein is supplied only from meat, it will be lacking in sulphurated amino acids, and this can hinder absorption of other amino acids.

To have a balanced food intake, an adult should eat 1 gram of meat per kilo of their weight, with a minimum of 60 grams per day for a woman and 70 for a man.

People doing sport to a high level and who want to increase the size of their muscles can go up to 1.5 grams per kilo of weight of proteins, as long as they drink plenty of liquids.

MEALS	FOODS	ANIMAL PROTEINS	VEGETABLE PROTEINS
Breakfast	150 ml of milk 60 g of wholemeal bread	5	5
Lunch	150 g fish 150 g wholemeal pasta 50 g yoghurt	20	5
Dinner	200 g lentils 30 g cheese 60 g wholemeal bread	3	18 5
		33 g	33 g

In practical terms, a person who weighs sixty-six kilos (145 pounds) should eat about 33 grams (0.106 ounces) of animal proteins and 33 grams of vegetable proteins a day, and these can be in the proportions given in the table above.

These proteins should represent 15 % of the daily food intake. To help you in your choices you can refer to the following table:

FOODS CONTAINING PROTEINS		
	ANIMAL PROTEINS	VEGETABLE PROTEINS
Average Concentration	Beef veal Mutton Pork Poultry Pork products Fish Processed cheeses	Soya beans Wheat germ Seaweed Grilled peanuts Lentils White beans Almonds
Large Concentration	Eggs Milk *Fromage frais* (soft cream cheeses)	Oat flakes Wholemeal bread Over 70 % cacao content chocolate Whole rye Wholemeal pasta Brown rice Walnuts Lentils

Food which is lacking in proteins can have serious consequences for the body: muscle wastage, healing difficulties, fallen uterus, etc.

If you have too much protein, however, gout can occur as the protein residues remain in the body and are transformed into uric acid. This is why you are advised to drink a lot to get rid of these residues.

It must nevertheless be noted the proteins are indispensable for good health and that even eating large quantities of them is not a difficulty unless you have serious kidney malfunction.

It must be noted also that they are generally associated with fats (lipids) in foods and often with saturated fats which must, unfortunately, be eaten with great prudence.

2. Glucides (carbohydrates)

These used to be called "hydrocarbons" because the are made of molecules of carbon, oxygen and hydrogen. Glucides (from the Greek word glukus, meaning "sweet") are also commonly grouped under the general term of "sugars".

a. Classification of glucides according to the complexity of their molecules (chemical formula)

Glucides with only one molecule (oligosaccharids)

– glucose, which is found in honey and in small quantities in fruit
– fructose, found mainly in fruit
– galactose, found in milk.

Glucides with two molecules (disaccharids)

– saccharose, which is none other than white sugar (castor or lumps) which is extracted from beet or from sugar cane (glucose + fructose);
– lactose (glucose + galactose), which is the sugar that is found in the milk of mammals;
– maltose (glucose + glucose), which is taken from malt, usually in beer or maize.

Glucides with more than two molecules (polysaccarides)

– glycogen, found in animal liver;
– starch, made up of a great many molecules of glucose, which is found in:
  • cereals: wheat, maize, rice, rye, barley, oats;
  • root vegetables: potatoes, yams
  • pulses: chick peas, dry beans, lentils, soya.

Some writers also include cellulose, hemicellulose, pectin from fruit and gums in this category, but actually these glucides cannot be assimilated during digestion and therefore do not contribute energy to the body. They should rather be classified as fibres.

For a long time glucides were only studied according to this classification (founded on their molecular structure), and put into two categories, **"simple sugars"** and **"complex sugars"**:

– **simple sugars** (one or two molecule glucides) and which it was thought needed little digestive transformation and were rapidly absorbed in the small intestine, were called **"fast sugars"**

– **complex sugars** which are formed from starch and which it was thought needed a long time to digest because of the complexity of their molecules, were called **"slow sugars"**. It was thought that they took longer to assimilate in the digestive system.

This classification of glucides into "fast" and "slow" sugars is completely out-of-date now and was in fact erroneous (see the frame below)

"Slow" and "Fast" sugars: an erroneous distinction

Most nutritionists and other dieticians today continue, without sanction, to pass on old-fashioned concepts of "slow" and "fast" sugars"

Professor Slama, a diabetics specialist, never lets an opportunity pass to remind us forcefully that glucides can only be classified according to their glycaemic importance.

Experience has shown that absorption of any kind of glucide (with single or multiple molecules) takes place about twenty to twenty-five minutes after eating.

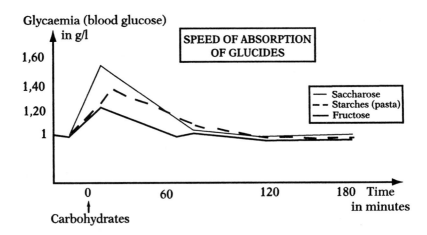

This false classification of glucides is still unfortunately used as a departure point for many of the dietary approaches, especially in sports nutrition, where it is still Gospel.

b. What is glycaemia?

Glucose can really be considered as the body's "fuel", and it effectively comes from two sources.

It is either synthesised by the body, which produces it from its reserve fat; or it results from the metabolism of glucides. In both cases without or without reserves (in the form of glycogen), glucose passes through the blood. This is why glycaemia can indicate the level of glucose in the blood.

The level of glycaemia before a meal is usually 1 gram per litre of blood (or 5.5 mmoll).

This is the biological parameter, amongst others, which is checked by your doctor when he asks for the results of your blood test.

When a glucide is absorbed on an empty stomach the variation in the level of blood glucose can be studied.

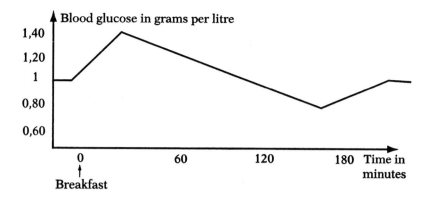

In the first stage, after eating on an empty stomach, glycaemia increases according to the kind of glucide ingested, until it reaches a maximum level which is called the "glycaemic peak". The pancreas, which plays an essential role in the functioning of the metabolism, will then secrete a hormone called insulin, which fulfils the purpose of chasing glucose from the blood to enable it to enter the cells which need it.

This is how in the second stage under the effect of the insulin the level of glycaemia falls.

In the third stage, glycaemia returns to normal.

c. Glycaemic index

Therefore, it is better to base the study of carbohydrates on the high or low rate of increase in glycaemia they induce rather than upon the carbohydrate assimilation rate.

Our concern then is with the 'glycaemic peak' of each carbohydrate eaten, that is to say its capacity to cause hyperglycaemia, as defined by the glycaemic index elaborated by Professor Crapo in the United States in 1976.

This glycaemic index in fact corresponds to the area of the triangle of the hyperglycaemic curve produced by the food tested. An index of 100 has been arbitrarily attributed to glucose and the index of other carbohydrates is therefore calculated by the following ratio:

$$\frac{\text{area of the triangle of the carbohydrate tested}}{\text{area of the triangle of the glucose}} \times 100$$

69

The glycaemic index will be all the higher if the hyperglycaemia caused by the tested carbohydrate is itself high.

Most scientists therefore recognise today that classification of carbohydrates must be made in accordance with their capacity to cause hyperglycaemia as defined by the glycaemic index concept.

In this book we will gradually see that this notion of the glycaemic index is fundamental. In fact, it is this that will enable us to explain not only plumpness, and even more so the cause of obesity, but also many of the problems of tiredness and lack of energy that worry our contemporaries in general and in particular women.

This is why, to simplify things, I propose to classify carbohydrates into two categories: "good carbohydrates" (those with a low glycaemic index) on the one hand, and "bad carbohydrates" (those with a high glycaemic index) on the other.

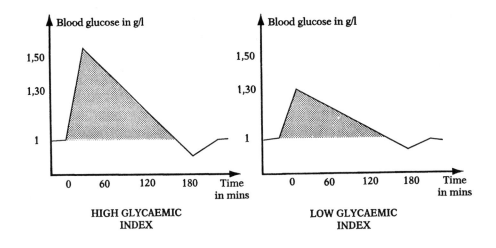

d. Bad carbohydrates (or glucides)

These are all carbohydrates which when eaten trigger a big increase in glucose in the blood and consequently provoke hyperglycaemia.

70

These are notably carbohydrates with a glycaemic index above fifty, which is the case with white sugar in all its forms, pure or combined with other nourishment (drinks, desserts, sweets, etc.), but also and above all industrially refined carbohydrates (bread, white pasta and white rice).

It will also be shown that some common consumer products such as potatoes and maize belong to these "bad carbohydrates". These have an even higher glycaemic index if they have undergone industrial processing (starches and potato flakes, corn flakes, pop-corn, etc.), or if they have been transformed by cooking (mashed potatoes, potatoes baked with grated cheese – *gratin dauphinois*).

Glycaemic Index Table

CARBOHYDRATES with high glycaemic index (bad carbohydrates)		CARBOHYDRATES with low glycaemic index (good carbohydrates)	
Maltose	110	Wholemeal bread or bread with bran	50
Glucose	100	Wholegrain rice	50
Baked potatoes	95	Peas	50
Very white bread	95	Wholegrain cereals without sugar	50
Mashed potatoes	90	Oat flakes	40
Honey	90	Fresh fruit juice (without sugar)	40
Carrots	85	Wholemeal rye bread	40
Cornflakes, popcorn	85	Wholewheat pasta	40
Sugar (sucrose)	75	Red kidney beans	40
White bread	75	Dried peas	35
Refined cereals with sugar	70	100 % stoneground wholemeal bread	35
Chocolate bars	70	Milk products	35
Boiled potatoes		Dried beans	30
Biscuits	70	Lentils	30
Corn (maize)		Chickpeas	30
White rice	70	100 % stoneground wholewheat pasta	30
Brown bread	65	Fresh fruit	30
Beetroot	65	Fruit preserve (without sugar)	25
Bananas	60	Dark chocolate (over 60 % cocoa)	22
Jam	55	Fructose	20
Non-wholewheat pasta	55	Soya	15
		Green vegetables, tomatoes, lemon, mushrooms	< 15

e. *Good carbohydrates*

Unlike the carbohydrates previously discussed, these are carbohydrates that give rise to a modest or even tiny release of glucose in the organism. They thereby lead to a smaller increase in glycaemia. This is the case of all raw cereals (unrefined flours), wild rice, and many starches and dried vegetables such as lentils, peas and beans.

Fruit and all green vegetables (leeks, cabbages, lettuces, green beans, etc.) can be added to this, and these are also recognised for their richness in fibres.

f. *Hyperglycaemia and insulin*

As we have seen previously, when absorption of a carbohydrate is at its highest point (glycaemic peak), the pancreas secretes insulin to reduce the glycaemia, as though chasing the glucose from the blood. The quantity of insulin produced will necessarily be in relation to the level of the glycaemia; hyperglycaemia therefore leads to hyperinsulinism in most cases.

We will come back to this idea later in greater detail as it is also fundamental to a good understanding of most metabolic phenomena and their consequences, notably weight gain

3. Lipids (or fats)

Fats have been the object of a veritable psychosis in the last few years in our societies. In the United States, behaviour towards them has almost become paranoid. For centuries they were the most sought after foods and the best loved, but today fat has become the main object of reproach and consequently it is this that is most often excluded from diets.

Traditional dietetics in fact made it responsible for obesity because it contains a lot of calories. It was also shown that through the bias of cholesterol it was responsible for most

72

cardio-vascular illnesses. It is now even accused of being an important contributing factor to some cancers.

We will come back to these sociological and epidemiological considerations in detail in a chapter devoted to hyper-cholesterolemia.

This chapter is of a technical nature, so we will only consider the subject here as realistically and objectively as possible.

Lipids, or reserve fats, are complex molecules which are more usually called fatty bodies. They are usually classified according to their sources:

– *lipids of animal origin:* these are fats contained in meat, fish, butter, milk products and cheese, eggs, etc.
– *lipids of vegetable origin:* these are oils (olive, sun-flower, etc.) and margarine.

It would however be better to classify lipids according to their chemical formulæ. Then two kinds can be seen:

– **saturated fatty acids**, found in meat, pork products, eggs, milk products (milk, butter, cream, cheeses), palm oil, etc.
– **mono-unsaturated and poly-unsaturated fatty acids**, which are fats which stay liquid at room temperature (sunflower oil, olive oil, rapeseed oil, etc.), although some of them can be hardened by hydrogenation (as in manu-facture of margarine);
– **unsaturated fats** from fish, goose and duck.

Consumption of lipids in the food intake is important or even essential as:

– they provide energy which can be stored in the form of reserve fats and can be available at any time to supply the body with glucose;
– they are at the origin of the formation of membranes and cells;
– they come into the composition of tissues and particularly of the nervous system;

- they help the manufacture of hormones and prostaglandins;
- they form the basis for the manufacture of bile salts;
- they carry the liposoluble vitamins, A, D, E, and K;
- they are the only sources of what are called "essential" fatty acids: linoleic and alphalinolenic acid
- some fatty acids play a preventive role in cardio-vascular pathology.

a. Lipids and obesity

Fats are the greatest energy providers, that is why they are public enemy number one for low calorie diets.

But, as we shall find out later, it is less the quantity of energy that is to be blamed as far as food is concerned than bad eating habits which destabilise the metabolism and lead to the building of reserve fats. We will see that it is hyperglycaemia which, through hyperinsulinism contributes in great measure to the abnormal storing of fat excesses arising from lipids (lipogenesis).

b. Lipids and cholesterol

The correlation between the excessive consumption of fats and the level of blood cholesterol (which is responsible for cardio-vascular illnesses) has in fact been shown. But this statement would not be complete without a certain reserve, as total cholesterol can be subdivided into two types of cholesterol: "good" and "bad".

The ideal would be to maintain a total cholesterol level below or equal to 2 grams per litre, and in which the proportion of "good" cholesterol would be as high as possible.

What you have to know is that all fats do not raise the "bad" cholesterol. On the contrary, there are even some which have a tendency to lower it noticeably. This is what we shall look at in more detail in the chapter devoted to hypercholesterolemia and to cardio-vascular risks.

74

This is why we should, to be accurate, classify fats into three new categories.

Fats which increase cholesterol

These are saturated fatty acids that are principally found in meat, pork products, milk and whole milk products, butter and some cheeses.

Excessive consumption of saturated fats can lead to an increase in the blood cholesterol level which may predispose to cardio-vascular problems. Many studies have in addition tended to consider the over-indulgence in saturated fats as a risk factor in the appearance of some cancers.

Fats which have little influence on cholesterol

These are those found in poultry, crustaceans and eggs.

Fats which lower cholesterol and prevent arterial problems

These are unsaturated fatty acids, that are mainly found in oils (except palm oil), oilseeds and fish, and also in goose and duck fat (*foie gras*, duck *confits*, etc.)

Amongst these the following may be mentioned:
• *Mono-unsaturated fatty acids*, especially oleic acid from olive oil, which has the property of lowering total cholesterol and increasing "good cholesterol". These have the advantage of being chemically stable;
• *Poly-unsaturated fatty acids*, which are found notably in sunflower, maize and rapeseed oils and which lower total cholesterol. They are rich in essential fatty acids but have the drawback of being easily oxidised. These poly-unsaturated fatty acids when oxidised become just as bad for the arteries as a saturated fatty acid.

In the same way, chemical changes undergone by some vegetable fats when they solidify (become margarine) seem to change their properties.

c. Essential fatty acids

Linoleic acid and alpha-linolenic acid (which used to be grouped together under the name of vitamin F) merit special attention here insofar as their presence is indispensable in the food intake.

It has been effectively demonstrated in the last few years that these fatty acids have a prime role in the make-up of brain cell membranes and in the development of the nervous system. This means that brain functions of people who are deficient in these acids, especially when they are very young, can be compromised.

It has also been shown that their absence can be an important factor in the development of the most serious illnesses of the metabolism which affect the populations of industrialised societies, and principally all those illnesses which can be attributed to deficiency of the immunity defence system.

Bad eating habits nowadays as well as the doubtful nature of the products that we have at our disposal, especially when they are refined, are probably the reason for these deficiencies. Linoleic acid which is found in sunflower, maize and grapeseed oils lowers the risk of cardio-vascular disease.

Deficiency in linoleic acid can lead to difficulties in growth and to changes in cells which alter the skin, mucous and endocrinal glands and the sexual organs. The recommended daily dose is 10 grams, which can for example be obtained by eating 20 grams a day of sunflower, maize or Soya oil.

Alpha-linolenic acid, found in large quantities in rapeseed, walnut and wheat germ oils, is particularly important for the biochemistry of the nervous system. Deficiency can lead to a change in learning ability, anomalies in neuro-transmission, increased risk of thrombosis and lower alcohol tolerance. The daily recommended dose is 2 grams. This

76

amount can be got from daily consumption of 25 grams of rapeseed oil.

No oil can in isolation give a correct balance of oleic, linoleic and alpha-linolenic acids. Therefore you should mix (or alternate) two or three of the following different oils in your salad dressings: olive oil, sunflower oil, rapeseed oil.

d. Daily intake of lipids (fats)

Daily consumption of fats, in all their forms, should not represent more than 30 % of food intake. In France at present it is at least 45 % (two-thirds of which are composed of saturated fats).

The ideal would to be to spread the fat ration out by eating 25 % saturated fats (meat, pork products, butter, whole milk products), 50 % mono-unsaturated fatty acids (goose fat, olive oil) and 25 % poly-unsaturated fatty acids (fish, sunflower oil, rapeseed oil, maize oil, etc.).

We will return to this advice in greater detail later.

Non-energy providing nutrients

The fact that some nutrients do not provide energy does not mean that they have no nutritional value.

On the contrary: but because they do not provide energy this has led many in our society to neglect them, whereas their food role is vital.

1. Food Fibres

Our ancestors ate fibres without realising it. We strangely only discovered them a short time ago when we came to see that we were not eating enough of them.

Food fibres, which are actually found mostly in carbohydrates with a low and often very low glyceamic index are substances of vegetable origin, usually combined with other nutrients. They are defined as *"vegetable residues which resist enzyme action in the small intestine, but are partially liquefied by the bacterial flora of the colon"*.

These are substances of vegetable origin with a chemical formula made up of complex carbohydrates. They are sometimes called "indigestible carbohydrates". Some food packaging includes them in the total carbohydrate count. But it is wrong to include them under this heading as they cannot be digested and do not increase glycaemia.

a) The various types of fibre

There are two kinds of fibre which each have very different properties:
– Insoluble fibres
These are called cellulose, and most of them are hemi-cellulose and lignin. They are found in fruit, vegetables, cereals and pulses.
– Soluble fibres
These are pectin (from fruits), gums (from pulses), alginates from seaweed (asgar, guar, carragahen) and hemicellulose from barley and oats.

b) The effects of fibres

Insoluble fibres when they swell up with water like sponges, speed up the evacuation of the stomach, and also increase the volume and moisture content of the faeces, which helps in their expulsion.

Their prime role is therefore as an excellent prevention of constipation (when they are associated with a high liquid intake). But they also contribute to lowering the blood cholesterol level and even more, to preventing the appearance of bile stones. Finally, they help to prevent colon and rectum cancer, which in France still are the cause of 25 000 deaths a year!

Once upon a time phytic acid in cereal was accused of interfering in the absorption of calcium. It was even said that "wholemeal bread led to decalcification". Modern science has shown that this is not the case, above all if the bread is made with yeast and traditional methods are followed in making it (no speeding up of the kneading process).

Fibres do not interfere with the absorption of vitamins or oligo-elements either, especially as foods which are rich in fibres (fruits, pulses, vegetables) often contain a good many micro nutrients which are indispensable for proper functioning of the body.

Soluble fibres, by absorbing a great amount of water, turn into a thick "jelly" with many properties. Because of high volume, it fully fills the stomach, which makes you feel full before you have eaten a lot. Therefore, without having absorbed calories, the feeling of hunger disappears more quickly.

It slows absorption of carbohydrates and fats and therefore when foods rich in soluble fibres have been eaten glycaemia rises less than it would with an identical amount of carbohydrates. Insulin secretion is therefore lower and as this hormone facilitates fat storage, less weight is gained. To sum up, a sufficient ration of soluble fibres will help slimming if you need to lose weight.

In the same way, fibres help to improve the diabetic's balance, as they lower the level of glycaemia. Diabetics should therefore choose to eat carbohydrates that are rich in soluble fibres (and especially fruit, haricot beans, lentils), which have a lower glycaemic index.

As fibres lower the blood cholesterol level, they constitute a protective factor against cardio-vascular disease. This is even more the case as some foods which are rich in fibres

79

(vegetables, raw fruits and oilseeds) contain anti-oxidants (vitamins C and E, beta-carotene) which also protect the walls of the arteries.

This beneficial action on blood fats also applies to tri-glycerides. We can only deplore the fact that in all the industrialised countries, and above all in the United States, the consumption of fibres has been abnormally lowered.

In France at the moment only 17 grams of fibre a day is consumed per inhabitant, whilst the daily dose should be 40 grams. A minimum of 30 grams should be adhered to.

As for the Americans, they presently consume less than 10 grams, which is a catastrophe.

2. Water

The liquid content of the body is 45 to 60 % of the weight of an adult individual in good health.

People can survive for weeks without food but only a few days without water. They can lose their glycogen and fat reserves and half of their proteins without being in real danger, but 10 % dehydration only can cause noticeable tiredness.

Everyone knows that the water lost in urine, breathing and sweating, and even in the faeces has to be replaced. The amount lost in these functions is about two and a half litres a day.

It is replaced by:

– drinks: 1.5 litres a day (water, skimmed milk, fruit juice, tea, soup, etc.);
– water contained in solid foods (bread for example contains 35 % water);
– water from the metabolism, that is to say, water produced by the various chemical processes of the body.

If you drink enough, the urine should be clear. If it is too yellow this is a sign that the amount of drinks is quite insufficient.

3. Mineral salts and oligo-elements

Mineral salts are essential substances for human life. They are actively present in various metabolic functions and in the electrochemistry of the nervous system and the muscles, as well as in the formation of such structures as bones and teeth. Some minerals also have the role of catalysts in many of the biochemical reactions of the body.

Minerals can be classified in two groups:
– those which are needed in relatively large quantities by the body: these are macro-elements;
– those which are only found in minute amounts: these are oligo-elements.

These substances act as catalysts for the biochemical reactions of the body. These are in a way the intermediaries which activate the work of the enzymes, and in their absence chemical reactions cannot take place. They are therefore indispensable even if they only act in infinitely small quantities.

Some oligo-elements have been known for a long time. Iron is one example, and its influence on health was noticed from the times of Antiquity, even though it was not known how it worked.

But most of them have been discovered recently, during research being done on what is often called "social illnesses", for example lack of vitality, or more precisely, tiredness.

Oligo-elements are the metals or metalloids present in the body in very low quantities (coming from the Greek *oligos* meaning "small").

The two questions which remain to be resolved concerning the oligo-elements are related to their quantity and their quality.

Agricultural land is becoming impoverished in oligo-elements. Because of intensive industrial exploitation through use of massive amounts of chemical fertiliser and phosphates and the fact that natural fertiliser of animal origin has not been replaced. This is particularly true as far as manganese deficiency is concerned.

MINERAL SALTS	OLIGO-ELEMENTS
Sodium	Iron
Potassium	Iodine
Calcium	Zinc
Phosphorus	Copper
Magnesium	Manganese
	Fluoride
	Chomium
	Selenium
	Cobalt
	Molybdenum

Vegetables grown on this impoverished land are themselves poor in oligo-elements. Even the animal world is effected. You only have to add zinc to cow food in some cases for them to be able to start having calves again. Without zinc procreation cannot occur.

As our food is more and more deficient in oligo-elements, we are consequently lacking in them ourselves. Many specialists believe that this is the basis for many of the pathological problems we find at the end of the XXth Century.

There are only two solutions, either go backwards, and that is what organic farming is successfully proposing, or add supplements to our food, but this could only be a transition period before a return to a kind of farming which is closer to our natural needs.

4. Vitamins

Throughout the centuries the appearance of diseases clearly related to bad feeding have been noticed in special circumstances (city sieges, famines, sea journeys).

This was the cause of bleeding gums caused by scurvy, bone diseases due to rickets, paralysis and oedemas due to beriberi and skin lesions due to pellagra.

We had to wait until the end of the XIXth century and even the beginning of the XXth before this imbalance was linked to the absence of indispensable substances called vitamins in the food.

Apart from the historical cases mentioned above, the existence of these essential nutrients was unknown, as the food eaten by humanity generally contained enough of them for notable deficiencies not to occur.

With the changes in food habits in the last few decades, generalisation of consumption of refined products (white sugar, white flour, white rice), development of intensive agriculture and its corollary, industrial processing, new deficiencies are found more and more frequently, or at least subsidiary deficiencies in some vitamins.

Vitamins could be defined as necessary organic compounds small quantities of which are needed to maintain life, stimulate growth and enable humanity to reproduce like most other animals.

They come from several sources. Non-fat meat from animals, especially offal (liver and kidneys) is one source which contains large concentrations.

Seeds, such as pulses, walnuts, hazelnuts, as well as whole cereals are also rich in vitamins. Roots and tubers (potatoes) are less rich. As for fruits and green vegetables, their content is patchy. The content may vary according to the kind of soil and also according to the weather and the storage conditions or even cooking conditions if they are cooked.

It is easy enough to lump all vitamins together, but they are nonetheless, because of their structure and the way they

83

act, a varied group. They should, then, be considered separately. They may however be classified into two groups: liposoluble (fat soluble) vitamins on the one hand and hydrosoluble (water soluble) vitamins on the other.

a. Liposoluble vitamins

There are four liposoluble vitamins: A, D, E and K. They are generally associated with fatty foods when they occur naturally: butter, cream, vegetable oils, fats and some vegetables.

The common properties of liposoluble vitamins are the following:

- they are stable when heated and do not even deteriorate in cooking;
- they are stored in the body and notably in the liver, which means that a deficiency takes a long time to become obvious;
- they can be toxic if they are taken in excessive quantities (especially vitamins A and D).

b. Hydrosoluble vitamins

As indicated by their name, these vitamins are soluble in water and can therefore be eliminated in the urine should they be taken in excess. Even though each of them has its own properties it has become clear that they are intimately linked by the various cell reactions that they are involved in.

The main hydrosoluble vitamins are the following:

- vitamin C: ascorbic acid;
- vitamin B1: thiamine;
- vitamin B2: ribioflavin;
- vitamin PP: niacin;
- vitamin B5: pantothenic acid;
- vitamin B8: biotin;

– vitamin B9: folic acid (folacin);
– vitamin B12: cyanocobalamin.

Like the oligo-elements, vitamins are therefore catalysts for many biochemical reactions. We are now quite familiar with the consequences of their absence as, in most cases, the symptoms are evident.

What is less well-known however are the conditions of their inter-dependence and the exact consequences arising from deficiencies in them.

But what we already know is very important. In the light of this knowledge which is being added to daily from new observation it is difficult not to ask further questions. That is why we are led to ask the right questions, and to see that they mostly lead to answers.

We will discover in the following chapters that a little stoutness and to a greater extent, obesity, are more the result of a de-stabilisation of the metabolism than of too rich a diet, as we have too often been led to believe.

We will particularly see that drastically reducing the amounts of your food as the calorie theory diets do, can only lead to an aggravation of deficiencies in minerals and vitamins for which our modern food is already responsible.

We shall be even more surprised to learn that paradoxically it is these erroneous reductions in calories that through one frustration after another lead in the long term to the obesity which is so characteristic of industrialised societies and especially the United States.

It is these various realisations concerning food change and pollution that we will be considering in greater depth in the following chapters and from this we will come to learn everything that must be done, if not to avoid, at least to considerably limit their bad effects.

As I told you right at the beginning of this book, the interest of this technical chapter is capital. In any case, it is indispensable to understanding the Method generally and especially to understanding the chapter which follows. Now that you know the nutritional composition of foods, you will finally be able to understand why you get fatter and how you can really and finally eat yourself slim.

CHAPTER IV

WHY DO WE GAIN WEIGHT?

Traditional dietetics, still unrelentingly based on the calorie theory with all its restrictions, would have you believe that if you gain weight, excluding possible hereditary factors, it is because you eat too much.

You know that this untrue, as everyone who has tried to slim by cutting down the amount of food they eat has not only failed to lose excess weight on a long-term basis but has very often found that they often regained and put on weight over and above their initial weight after a few months

Once again, it is not excess energy from food that is to blame for reserve fat but, as we shall see in detail in this chapter, the nature of the food consumed, that is to say its nutritional characteristics.

Once again, I would like to recommend that you read this chapter very carefully even if, as for the previous one, it is of a somewhat technical nature. It would be regrettable if you were to go straight to the chapter on the Method without having understood the real reason for putting on weight.

To explain the question "why do we gain weight" we must look at the level of glycaemia rise and its consequences in facilitating storage of fats.

We previously explained that the body's fuel is glucose. The permanent reservoir that all organs requiring glucose dip into to function (brain, heart, kidneys, muscles, etc.) is the blood.

We have seen that this "reservoir" theoretically contains an amount corresponding to 1 gram of glucose per litre of blood. In effect, the body has two means of obtaining the glucose it needs and maintaining the level in its reservoir at 1 gram per litre of blood.

The first method of obtaining glucose is to manufacture it. The body is in fact capable of making glucose at any time from the reserve fats stored in the fatty tissue.

In cases of dire necessity, it can even make glucose from the lean tissues, that is to say from proteins present in the muscles.

The second way of obtaining glucose is by eating foods belonging to the glucide (carbohydrate) family, for instance, sugars, fruit and other starches (see Chapter III of Part I).

We know that when a carbohydrate is eaten, the body transforms it (we say metabolises it) into glucose during the digestive process, that is all excepting the fructose.

But before being stored in the body in the form of glycogen, the glucose from digestion passes through the blood stream.

In other words, when a carbohydrate is eaten, the corresponding glucose produced will suddenly increase glycaemia.

When you eat a fruit, a sweet or starches, blood glycaemia will suddenly rise above its normal level (which as we know is 1 gram per litre of blood).

You might, for example, go from 1 gram to 1.2 grams when you eat a fruit, or to 1.70 grams by eating potatoes. The sudden increase in glycaemia, through the absorption of a carbohydrate, is called hyperglycaemia.

As soon as you go well over the level of 1 gram of glucose per litre of blood you become hyperglycaemic. On the other hand, when glycaemia becomes too low (around 0.5 gl) it is said that one is hypoglycaemic (see the graph below).

As we saw in the previous chapter, hyperglycaemia arising from consumption of a carbohydrate is related to its glycaemic index.

Thus, if we eat a fruit with a very low glycaemic index (30), hyperglycaemia will be very low. If on the other hand we eat a sweet (glycaemic index of 75), or a baked potato (glycaemic index of 95), hyperglycaemia will be high and the curve could reach 1.75 grams, for example.

The normal level being 1 gram per litre, as soon as you go above this, a control mechanism will be triggered. This is governed by a very important organ called the pancreas, which secretes insulin.

The main property of this hormone is to lower glycaemia by causing the glucose to enter the organs which need it. Its second function is to aid storage of reserve fats.

So, as soon as blood glycaemia rises above 1 gl, the pancreas secretes insulin to bring the curve back to normal.

In the same way, as soon as the level falls abnormally low (hypoglycaemia) the body finds a way to raise the blood glucose level again in order to regain a balance.

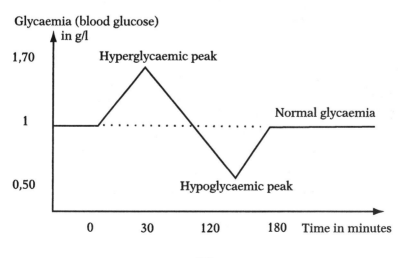

Normally, the amount of insulin made by the pancreas in order to lower glycaemia is directly proportional to the level of glycaemia.

For example, if you eat a fruit which only creates low level hyperglycaemia, the pancreas will send very little insulin out to lower this glycaemia level as the compensation involved is very small.

However, if you eat something sweet which sets off high glycaemia, the pancreas has to send a big dose of insulin into the blood to re-establish glycaemia level.

In every scenario, the glucose which has been hunted out of the blood by the insulin will be stored in the liver (in the form of glycogen), or else used by the organs that need it, such as the brain, the kidneys or the red blood corpuscles.

But we now know that if someone has a tendency to put on weight, and even more so when they have a tendency to obesity, it is because they are suffering from a pancreatic malfunction. This means that when they have high hyperglycaemia their pancreas will secrete an excessive dose of insulin. It is then said that they are suffering from hyperinsulinism.

It has been scientifically proved that hyperinsulinism is responsible for abnormal build-up of reserve fats.

To better understand this phenomenon let us do two experiments: the first when a person with a tendency to fatness eats a slice of buttered bread.

First experiment

We will make the subject eat 100 grams of white bread on which we spread 30 grams of butter. The bread will be metabolised into glucose and the butter into fatty acid, both of which will pass through the blood stream (see diagram 1, p. 92).

The white bread is a glucide (carbohydrate) with a high glycaemic index (70) which therefore results in high hyperglycaemia (about 1.70 grams).

To lower this glycaemia, the pancreas will therefore have to secrete a certain amount of insulin. But, as we are dealing with a malfunctioning pancreas, the amount of insulin will be disproportionate to the normal amount (see diagram 2, p. 92), and it is this hyperinsulinism which will trigger abnormal storage of part of the fatty acids from the butter (see diagram 3 and 4, p. 92).

Second experiment

This time we will make the subject eat 100 grams of wholemeal bread upon which we will still spread our 30 grams of butter (see diagram 1, p. 93). The wholemeal bread having a lower glycaemic index (35) only low glycaemia results (about 1.20 grams). To lower this slight glycaemia, the pancreas will secrete only a small amount of insulin (see diagram 2, p. 93).

As hyperinsulinism does not arise when only a slight call is made on the pancreas it will only secrete the insulin dose necessary to make the low glycaemia fall (see diagram 3, p. 93).

As a consequence, the fatty acids in the butter will not be abnormally stored as there is no excess insulin (see diagram 4, p. 93).

Even though this experiment with the buttered bread is somewhat sketchy it is enough to make you understand the mechanism that leads to the building of reserve fat and hence excess weight.

In both cases our "guinea pig" ate the same thing: 100 grams of bread + 30 grams of butter. Why does the first one get fatter whereas the second one does not?

First Experiment

Eating 100 grams of white bread and 30 grams of butter

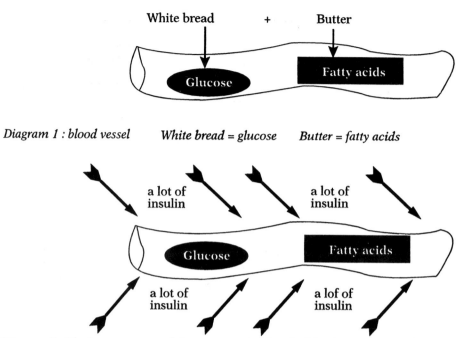

White bread   +   Butter

Glucose

Fatty acids

Diagram 1 : blood vessel   White bread = glucose   Butter = fatty acids

a lot of insulin   a lot of insulin

Glucose   Fatty acids

a lot of insulin   a lof of insulin

Diagram 2 : The large amount of glucose contained in the blood system sets off a high secretion of insulin, therefore hyperinsulinism

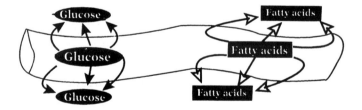

Diagram 3 : The insulin chases out the glucose from the blood but the excess glucose (hyoperinsulinism) takes with it a large part of the fatty acids

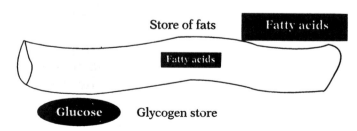

Store of fats   Fatty acids

Fatty acids

Glucose   Glycogen store

Diagram 4 : Glucose is stored in the form of glycogen.
The fatty acids are stored in reserve fats, hence weight gain

Second Experiment
eating 100 grams of wholemeal bread and 30 grams of butter

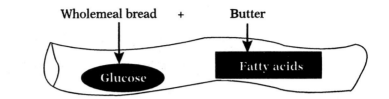

Diagram 1 : Blood vessel   *Wholemeal bread = glucose*   *Butter = fatty acids*

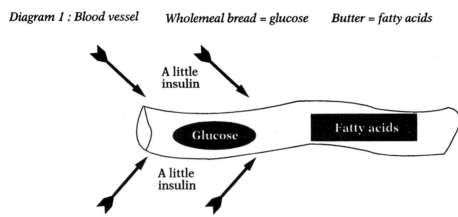

Diagram 2 : As there is only a little glucose present only a very small amount of insulin is secreted

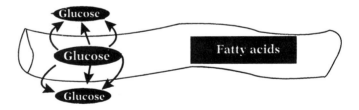

Diagram 3 : The small insulin secretion makes it possible to chase the glucose from the blood, but it is not enough to take the fatty acids with it

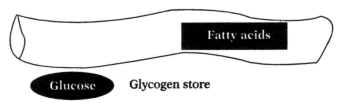

*Diagram 4 : Glucose is stored in the form of glycogen.
Fatty acids are not stored in the form of reserve fats, therefore no weight gain*

Because of the kind of bread, of course! The only explanation is the nutritional composition of the bread.

White bread is of course a refined food. Not only its fibres but also most of its proteins, vitamins, mineral salts and oligo-elements have been removed. This is the reason why its glycaemic index is high. Wholemeal bread on the other hand is a raw food in which all the original nutritional content remains, and especially the fibres and proteins. This is why its glycaemic index is low.

White bread induces high glycaemia and leads, therefore, to weight gain (storage of butter) through the action of hyperinsulinism. Wholemeal bread which for its part leads only to a low glycaemia, does not aid storage of the fatty acids from the butter as there will be no excessive secretion of insulin (hyperinsulinism).

We have thus demonstrated the fact that it is not the quantity of energy contained in foods (which is almost identical for these two kinds of buttered bread) which leads to weight gain.

It is the nature of the food eaten, that is to say, the nutritional content, which will lead or not to added weight.

There is no rise in weight in the first case because the glycaemic index of the bread is sufficiently low to avoid hyperinsulinism, which is the real trigger for weight gain.

But we have been very careful in describing this experiment to be specific about the fact that this was a subject suffering from pancreatic hyperinsulinism.

What distinguishes a thin from a fat person? If one of them gets fatter (the obese one) and is eating the same things (carbohydrates with high glycaemic level) it is because or hyperinsulinism. In this case, the balance between the amount of insulin secreted and the amount of carbohydrates ingested does not add up.

The person may not yet be aware of it, but will not fail

to notice soon if they continue to eat excessive amounts of bad carbohydrates.

At this stage we can also easily understand that fatness and even more so, obesity, are only the indirect consequences of too high a carbohydrate level in food with a high glycaemic index (too much white sugar, too much white flour, too many potatoes) in association with an intake of fats.

Excessive consumption of bad carbohydrates will in effect be turned into permanent hyperglycaemia, the consequence of which will be abnormal stimulation of the pancreas. The latter may at first be strong enough to withstand the bad treatment, for which it was not intended, for a few years, but will begin to show signs of fatigue. This is why people put on weight with age, fatness always being proportional to the development of the level of hyperinsulinism.

Glycaemic results of a meal

Some of my detractors let it be understood that the glycaemic index idea is only theoretical and emphasise that meals are usually made up of a number of foodstuffs amongst which carbohydrates have only relative importance. However, on the contrary, some studies have shown that the idea of a glycaemic index is still valid in the case of a more complicated meal. It certainly depends on the amount of carbohydrates absorbed, but also on the amounts of proteins and fibres eaten at the same time. There really is then a glycaemic result to a meal, and studies show that it is only slightly less than if the main carbohydrate of a meal had been eaten in isolation.

But over and above the idea of a glycaemic index, the level of insulin secretion has to be taken into account. It has even been shown that the amount of insulin triggered is always higher (except for haricot beans) when the glucide is eaten in a more complex meal than when it is taken in isolation by a person suffering from hyperinsulinism. This is the case with an obese person (and a diabetic not dependent upon insulin).

95

If you were fat as a child, your pancreas was already in a bad state when you landed on this earth, no doubt for hereditary reasons. And the bad food habits that you have adopted since (too many bad carbohydrates) have only aggravated the situation.

If today Western societies have a serious overweight and obesity problem it is because our fellow citizens have adopted diets in the last fifty years or so in which bad carbohydrates play too large a part.

In reality, we have been changing our food traditions for about one-hundred-and-fifty years. It is in fact since the first half of the XIXth century that new foods, all of them hyperglycaemic, have become widespread in Western societies: sugar, potatoes and white flours.

Sugar

Until the XVIth century, sugar was almost unknown in the Western world. It was sometimes eaten as a spice, the rarity of which made it extremely expensive, only available to the richest.

The discovery of the New World facilitated a relative development of sugar cane but transportation and refining costs still left it as a luxury product reserved for the few.

In 1780, sugar consumption was less than one kilo per year and per head of population. It was the discovery of the process of extracting sugar from beet in 1812 that gradually made sugar a widespread consumer product, and its price came down constantly.

Consumption statistics are as follows for France:

– 1800: 0.6 kilos per year and per head
– 1880: 8 kilos per year and per head
– 1900: 17 kilos per year and per head
– 1930: 30 kilos per year and per head

96

– 1965: 40 kilos per year and per head
– 1990: 35 kilos per year and per head

As we know, sugar is a carbohydrate with a high glycaemic index (75). Consumption of sugar leads to hyperglycaemia which has for a consequence the excessive stimulation of the pancreas.

We can therefore consider that the discovery of beet sugar greatly upset eating habits in our societies, to such an extent that it can be said that there has never been so radical a change in food habits in the history of mankind in such a short period of time.

The French can however rejoice in the fact that they are the lowest consumers of sugar in the Western world. The English eat 49 kilos per head a year, the Germans 52 kilos, and the world record has been achieved by the Americans with 63 kilos per head a year!

Potatoes

Some may believe that potatoes form part of the cultural heritage of old Europe. Nothing of the kind! They really began to spread only at the beginning of the XIXth century, after Parmentier suggested them as a substitute for wheat during the famine periods before the French Revolution.

After its discovery in Peru, in the middle of the XVIth century, the potato was only used to fatten pigs. It was then called the pig root and was usually viewed with great circumspection because it belongs to the botanical solonacia family, and most of the species is poisonous.

What is of interest to us today is to know that potatoes have one of the highest glycaemic indexes, as when there are baked it is higher than that of sugar.

Cooking methods are very important for potatoes, as they can bring out greater or lesser quantities of resistant starches (non-digestible). When potatoes are cooked in the oven, or mashed, the amount of resistant starch is low, and most of it is digested.

In addition, potatoes have a very mediocre interest as a food as, added to their excessive hyperglycaemic effect, their nutritional content after cooking is low (8 mg 100 of vitamin C and very little fibre). Their vitamin, mineral and oligo-element content is negligible also as it is found around the skin and is therefore systematically eliminated with peeling. Their value also decreases with prolonged storage.

Refined flours

Flour has always been sifted through a sieve. In the past it was roughly done, by hand, and given the cost (30 % wastage), it was only available to a few privileged people.

The masses only had the right to black bread and so the French Revolution made white bread one of its essential symbolic platforms.

However, it was not until 1870 with the discovery of the rolling mill that the price of refining flour came down substantially and it was possible to give their daily white bread to a greater number of people.

We now know that refined flour is lacking in any nutritional content: proteins, essential fatty acids, vitamins, mineral salts, oligo-elements, fibres.

Above all, we also know that refining a wheat flour increases its glycaemic index from 35 to 70, which thus turns it into a hyperglycaemic food.

In our societies (except for the Americans) we probably eat less bread today than a hundred years ago, but we eat more white flour: white pasta, sandwiches, pizzas, biscuits, various cakes, etc.

White rice and maize

White rice, as everyone knows, comes from Asia where the inhabitants generally eat it with vegetables with a high fibre, vitamin, mineral salt and oligo-element content and the glycaemic implications of white rice are reduced by these. Westerners, who invented the refining process, more often eat it with meat, that is, with saturated fats.

It must also be added that sticky rice, which is authentically Asian, even has (when it is white) a glycaemic index which is much lower than Western rice (especially American) the species of which have been selected for their productivity. In any case, this is a fourth carbohydrate with a high glycaemic index which has only recently been introduced into our modern food catalogue.

The same goes for maize. The varieties we eat in the West correspond to hybrid seeds which have been developed in laboratories, in the framework of agronomic research directed uniquely towards productivity.

The maize that was originally eaten by the American Indians has a glycaemic index which is much lower (about 30). It has been proved that the higher fibre content is what explains the difference.

This high level of soluble fibre content not only led to low glycaemia but it also enabled it to retain its moisture.

Hence, it will be understood that because of the absence of soluble fibres, modern maize requires a great deal of irrigation, which has the ecological consequences that we are aware of as far as depletion of the water table is concerned.

If we really want to understand the Western phenomenon of fatness and obesity, we only have to note the changes of food traditions in the modern world that have occurred in favour of hyperglycaemic foods (sugar, potatoes, flours, white rice) and to the detriment of low glycaemic index carbohydrates (green vegetables, lentils, beans, peas, raw cereals, fruit, etc.) which were the base of our nourishment in the old days.

You can also understand why all the agronomic research in the last few years has been geared solely towards productivity objectives, and this has been done to the detriment of the nutritional quality of the foods. In the case of cereals, for example, this impoverishment has been translated into higher glycaemic indexes, with the metabolic consequences of which we are aware.

When you look at the glycaemic index table (see Chapter III), it is very noticeable that modern food products are found in the left hand column (high glycaemic index) and the more traditional foods are found in the right hand column.

Changing traditional eating patterns in our Western societies correspond to the movement of the foods from the right-hand column to the left-hand column and therefore to the adoption of a nutritional model in which carbohydrates with a high glycaemic index predominate.

Since the beginning of the XIXth century, Western populations have progressively introduced more and more hyperglycaemic products into their menus. But even if their pancreas was beginning to give signs of fatigue, obesity was still very marginal. There are two explanations for this.

Firstly, because people at the time ate far more vegetables and pulses than today, and this contributed large amounts of fibres. We know that fibres have the effect of lowering glycaemia and limiting pancreatic secretion.

In addition, the glycaemic index of cereals (even partially refined) was much lower, as we have seen above, because of the lower productivity. Secondly, and above all, because people ate very little meat because they could not afford it. This means to say that their fat consumption was low.

We already know that to trigger weight gain two factors are necessary: hyperglycaemic food intake generating hyperinsulinism, on the one hand, and a hyperlipidic (rich in fats) food intake on the other.

For more than a century in our societies, food was only gradually becoming hyperglycaemic, as there were no major increases in fat intake. Hyperinsulinism did not have the opportunity manifest its consequences, but it did nevertheless exist. If fatness has rapidly become widespread, and if obesity has suddenly arisen in Western countries since the Second World War, it is because one of the triggering factors (excessive consumption of fats) has suddenly appeared.

With a higher standard of living, Western societies quickly changed their food habits, giving precedence to consumption of meat, therefore of fats, but also to bad carbohydrates (sugars, refined flours, potatoes, non-stick white rice, hybrid maize), and less vegetables and lentils, that is to say, less fibres.

America is, we might add, the worst example in this respect, to the extent to which it is there that they eat both the most hyperglycaemic foods, the most meat, and the least green vegetables. It therefore comes as no surprise that the USA holds the world record for obesity.

Over the centuries, it has always been noticed that the few fat people were always the privileged. For a long time it was thought that they were fat because they were rich and they therefore ate more than the others.

In fact, they did not eat more than the masses, but only differently, as they were able to eat sugar and refined flours, which were rare and expensive.

Paradoxically, in the United States, it is amongst the poor that we find the greatest proportion of obesity today, and that is simply because hyperglycaemic food as well as very fatty meat, have become much cheaper.

As I have pointed out several times, this chapter is very important to the understanding of the principles of the Method, a detailed explanation of which will follow.

101

Re-read it several times until you are sure to have understood why it is the kind of carbohydrate that will cause fat to be stored or not. To be able to slim and never put the weight on again it is imperative to understand why we get fat.

The hope that you have of getting rid of your extra fat for good is based on the fact that in this respect the human body is capable of a complete reversal. All the Americans who come to France are surprised to lose weight by eating traditional French cooking. In the same way, French adolescents who spend a summer in the USA generally come back a little plumper.

This means to say that it is the eating habits that one adopts that cause us either to gain weight or to lose it. And it is the quality of what we eat and not the quantity that is responsible for this.

If you exclusively eat the carbohydrates in the left-hand column, those with a high glycaemic index, you will get fat. If you chose for preference those in the right-hand column, there is every chance that you will begin to lose weight.

Here you see why the Method that I am proposing is based on food choices. It is not restrictive, as you know, but it is on the other hand, selective. It is by choosing the foods that are right, whatever their quantity, that you are going to be able to slim effectively and durably, and at the same time continue to eat with pleasure and even gastronomically.

If, after a few months of applying Phase I correctly, you do not seem to have lost that much weight, or have not lost enough, you must look elsewhere for possible causes of this resistance to slimming.

I would immediately rule out the cases of women whose weight is already nearly ideal but who, in spite of being normal, doggedly want to slim, and also those who mistake cellulite for fat.

102

Other possible factors could have an influence and be the cause and some these must be pointed out:

– some medicines can have a negative influence on the metabolism, such as tranquillisers, antidepressants, lethium, beta-blockers, cortisone and sugary tonics (see Chapter VII, Part II);

– stress (which will speak about later). Managing it with a relaxation method may be necessary to be able to attain the right weight loss;

– hormonal problems which appear in women before or at the time of the menopause, with or without medical treatment (see Part II);

– Bulimia, which needs behaviour therapy.

CHAPTER V

THE METHOD

When we see advertisements on the television for food products we are always surprised by the contrast between the persuasive arguments used, which vary depending upon whether it is for animal food or food for poor human beings.

When the product advertised is for our animal friends, the advertising message scenario is quite classic. First of all the breeder comes along, because the reference to a professional always adds credence. Then there is a close up of the animal, a dog for example, running around the countryside, to emphasise its great vitality. Then they do not fail to draw our attention to its glossy coat and bright eyes, signalling its excellent health.

Finally, the vet appears, and explains that if this animal is in this exceptionally good condition it is because its master feeds it with product X, and he, the scientist, has been able to verify its quality. He then lists all the indispensable nutrients that have been added to it: proteins, vitamins, mineral salts, oligo-elements and fibres.

Should, however, the advert be praising the merits of a food product which ordinary mortals may eat daily, the scenario is quite different. The accent is then put almost exclusively on the price, the packaging or even on the ways of preserving it.

In a well-known French television advert, when an unlucky

cyclist arrives late after his fellow travellers have selfishly emptied the soup bowl, he is immediately reassured that he won't have to go without as the recommended packaged brand only needs a few seconds to make up a soup "just like the old days".

A real/false replacement, and nobody will be concerned about its contents (sodium glutamate, sugars, modified starch, preservatives, etc.) or wonder about its almost total lack of nutrients.

When an advertising executive thinks up a message, his professional expertise will invariably lead him to call upon sensitive themes and thereby refer to symbols which are important in the subconscious mind of the public.

Given that, why bother to list the nutritional contents of a food and praise their merits if no-one is sensitive to this argument and if, in addition, no-one could care less?

For nearly half a century our society has progressively forgotten the importance that the nutrition factor could have, not only for our health, but also for our survival.

Dieticians have only emphasised the energy giving aspects of food, so the food industry has been able to concentrate exclusively on economic objectives, which has allowed a tremendous development in technology to take place.

Thinking has been transformed. Urbanisation, the organisation of society, working women and leisure activities have progressively modified the relationship of individuals to their food.

The extreme illustration of this is naturally the American model.

In the USA, the act of feeding has been reduced to the satisfaction of a physiological need. Eating is like going to the toilet – an obligation. With this attitude, why spend much money? This is why choices are made primarily according to price. The marketing answer of the fast food retailers was, therefore, to propose a meal at 99 cents. Less than a dollar.

Within the framework of the organisation of the working

day, lunch in America is never a consideration – take the comment in the film *Wall Street* "lunch is for wimps". Officially it does not exist.   This is why they eat walking down the street or on the edge of the desk.   For a born Frenchman, food belongs to quite another category.   Eating is part of the ritual of life, even if it is a means of survival, and it is above all a chance to have a good time, because eating is part and parcel of a hedonistic attitude which should not be denigrated – as it seems often to be in more puritanical societies.   Another film well illustrates the opposing attitude: "Babette's Feast".

Culinary and even gastronomic traditions are not simply folklore, they are a fundamental part of the culture in France. *La cuisine*, which is not simply cooking, is an art, with all its nuances, distinctive features and specific geographical differences.   *La cuisine* and regional and local produce are part of the heritage and every authentic French person unconsciously ensures their transmission from generation to generation.

Lunch time is therefore sacred and the necessary time is allocated to it.   In the provinces, offices, shops and administrations close their doors; most people go home to join their families.   Others meet up in cafeteria or canteens. This meal is an important part of living itself, and it is treated as a real institution.

The art of living is indissolubly linked to the art of the table.   It is for this reason that the French spend time and do not hesitate to spend money on it.

The French paradox

On 17 November 1991, the best known American television programme, "Sixty Minutes" devoted twenty minutes to an article entitled "The French Paradox".

This revealed that the French, who spend a great deal of their time at table, eat 30 % more fats than the Americans, do no exercise and drink ten times more wine, are in fact in much better health than the Americans.

Their average weight curve is below that of any other Western country and their level of risk of death by cardio-vascular diseases is the lowest in the world after Japan.

The CBS programme was in fact using the observations gathered by the World Health organisation within the frame-work of a study called "Monica".

How do the French manage to cut to a third the cardio-vascular risks in relation to the Americans, whilst doing the opposite of what is being recommended all over America as far as prevention is concerned?

Scientists, perplexed, had to recognise that they had found several explanations:

- the French take time to eat;
- they eat three meals a day;
- they eat structured meals (three courses) of varied composition;
- they eat more vegetables and fruit, so more fibres and vitamins;
- they eat good fats (olive oil, sunflower oil, goose and duck fat, and fish)
- they drink wine, especially red wine, and they do so regularly.

Since the launch of the concept of the "French Paradox", which brought about an increase in the consumption of wine and *fois gras* in the United States, more in-depth studies have been undertaken. They show that today the nutritional ideal which should be taken as a model is that which has always been applied around the Mediterranean and has always inspired the larger part of the South of France.

Does this mean that, given these international observations, the French can just pat themselves on the back without any changes in their eating habits?

The French situation is certainly quite satisfactory, if it is compared to that of the Americans, which is dramatic. But this does not mean, for all that, that it has not suffered quite severe deterioration for some time.

The statistics tell us that in fact the average weight of adolescents in France has quite noticeably risen in the last few years (about + 15 % in twenty years).

In addition, a couple of years ago the medical journal *Le Quotidien du Médicin* reported a study carried out amongst young army recruits. It showed that 25 % of them now have too high a cholesterol level, whereas this was true of only 5 % twenty years ago.

The French Paradox is therefore not being confirmed for the up and coming generation, and for good reasons. This is the only generation that has for the moment denied their origins and completely changed its eating habits. Under the pressure of advertising they have unreservedly adopted the North American model in which coke and hamburgers are the leading lights.

Amongst adults, classical food habits are resisting better, as they are rooted in tradition. However, they are undergoing a slow and undeniable degradation owing to the change in lifestyle, over-standardisation of the agro-food industry and the impact of advertising messages.

Well, when we analyse the elements of modern eating fashions, we see that they are similar to those of our American cousins: that is to say, hyperglycaemic. The foods which dominate meals in our society now are mainly:

- **white flours** in all their forms (white bread, Danish pastries, sandwiches, hot dogs, pizzas, biscuits, cakes, crackers, white pasta, refined cereals, etc.);
- **sugar**, in fruit juice substitutes and such things as coke, but also in various sweets and especially in the "snack" bars (Mars bars, Kit-Kat, etc.);
- **potatoes**, mostly in their worst disguises: chips, crisps and roast potatoes;
- **Westernised white rice** which leads to even higher gly-

caemia when it is boiled in deep water which is poured away afterwards [1].

In the past, people ate vegetables from the garden, even if it was only in the soup. Thus the corresponding consumption of fibres was on average 30 grams a day per head. Today it is 17 grams, whilst the daily consumption of fibres should be at least 30 to 40 grams.

This being said, let's come to the point. The Montignac Method, as we are going to see, makes it possible to achieve good management of your weight balance. It is not, however, only centred around slimming, and has other objectives in mind:

– to ensure effective cardio-vascular disease prevention;
– to renew maximum vitality;
– to re-integrate food into the context that it should never have left, that means sociable and gastronomic. Eating should remain, first and foremost a shared pleasure!

The Method I am proposing is simple. It will first consist of a realigning of your eating habits, in accordance with the general concept of the glycaemic indexes.

You will clearly understand from the previous chapter that, if you have a tendency to get fat it is because your pancreas is in bad condition and is secreting an excessive quantity of insulin.

The whole of the eating strategy that we are going to implement will therefore consist of firstly, avoiding foods with a high glycaemic index, and secondly, giving preference to those with a low glycaemic index, as well as carefully choosing your fats.

Once again, I would warn my female readers: it is abso-

---

1. When rice is boiled the soluble fibres are dissolved. When the water is thrown away, as it is in Western countries, this means you have got rid of the fibres and this therefore comes down to raising your glycaemic index. This is why the Asians, in their great wisdom, cook rice in a small amount of water so that they do not have to throw any away and thus preserve all the fibres.

lutely indispensable to read and understand the previous chapters to be able to take advantage of the principles of the Method.

Many of you have seen your figure become deformed through following low calorie diets which were necessarily restrictive and had a time limit.

With a low calorie diet, all the lost weight goes back on as soon as you start eating as before, and you regain and even add weight because of the frustrations you have put your body through.

With the Method that I propose, it is not a question of adopting a different way of eating for a short time and then going back to your old habits.

As there are no restrictions on the quantity you eat, you will learn to eat according to different principles and many aspects of these will be adopted on a lifetime basis.

The surplus weight that you so deplore stems from your bad eating habits, and especially from the fact that you eat too many bad carbohydrates (glucides) and bad fats (lipids). The new eating method you will adopt will necessarily be more varied, more harmonious and above all, better balanced. When you have achieved the hoped-for results, there will therefore be no reason for you to go back to the disorderly and unhealthy eating habits that you had before.

The very fact of going from the foods in the left-hand column to those in the right hand column of the table of glycaemic indexes should be enough to achieve a substantial weight loss. To do that, you will need time, probably several months. If you want to get quicker results, and above all enable your pancreas to "recover its health", more selective measures can be taken in the early stage. The Method is therefore split into two phases:

– Phase I, which is the period of rapid weight loss and renewed vitality;
– Phase II, which is the "cruising" period and which will continue indefinitely.

PHASE I

This will last from one to several months, according to the person concerned and their aims. This is the time needed to change food habits, give up the bad ones and adopt good ones ("good" carbohydrate and "good" fat choices). The body will in a way "cleanse" itself and some metabolic functions (pancreatic secretion) will not be over-worked so that they will return to normal.

This phase is easy to follow as quantities are not limited. For those who are "subscribers" to low calorie diets, it will even be a pleasure as they will finally be able to slim and to go back to eating at the same time.

PHASE I is, however, selective, in the sense that some foods will be excluded (bad carbohydrates, or eaten in a certain way at a particular time of day.

This phase is easy to put into practise even when, and particularly, if meals are eaten away from home.

The meals will be varied and the food balanced, rich in proteins, fibres, vitamins, mineral salts and oligo-elements. In general, Phase I does not cause frustration, as someone who assuages their hunger avoids the risk of a com-pensating with bulimia (bingeing). Happily, the good effects of the new way of eating can be seen on a daily basis.

But before going into the details of PHASE I, we should

112

go over a few general points, which though general are nevertheless fundamental.

Three meals a day

The rule of keeping to three meals a day may seem too simplistic to be mentioned. It is, however, of the greatest importance. In any case, it implies that a meal should never be missed and that snacking in the American fashion should naturally be avoided.

People who are afraid of getting fat are generally just those who take the risk of missing meals, especially lunch.

"Are you coming to lunch?", a secretary may ask her colleague.

"No", the latter replies, *"this evening I'm having dinner with friends, so you see, I'm being careful, watching my weight"*.

This illustrates a huge mistake that is made daily. Remember what we saw in the chapter on low calorie diets: the best way of getting fat is not to eat!

If you miss a meal your body will suffer withdrawal symptoms, panic and therefore be on the defensive when the next meal comes and will deliberately take advantage of it to create reserves. These reserves will then be even more substantial if the meal is a large one.

Order of importance of the three meals

When you get up in the morning, the stomach has theoretically been empty for at least eight or nine hours.

The first meal of the day, breakfast, should therefore be the biggest. This is what happened in the past. Today, it is the most neglected meal. For many people it comes down to a cup of coffee or tea, drunk on an empty stomach without the least bit of solid food.

This practice is naturally catastrophic on the metabolic level. Some may object, saying *"But in the morning, apart from the fact that I don't have time, the real problem is that I'm not hungry"*.

The answer is easy! If you are not hungry in the morning it is because you ate too much in the evening. It is a bit of a vicious circle.

You then have to as it were "prime the pump" one day by considerably reducing the evening meal (or even cutting it out). This may seem to contradict what was said in the previous paragraph, but it is a different problem.

Lunch should be normal, or at least big enough to take over from breakfast.

As to dinner, it should be as light as possible, and in any case as long as possible from bedtime, because the body reconstitutes its reserves during the night. Let us say more simply that the same food eaten in the evening will be more "fattening" than if it had been eaten in the morning or at lunch time.

We will return later to each of these three nutritional stages of the day, and each time we will explain what the ideal would be and what should be avoided.

You will, unfortunately, understand that most people in our societies do exactly the opposite.

Modern lifestyles have in fact lead us to create a hierarchy for the three meals which is exactly the opposite of what should be the case:

– breakfast is nothing, or only the lightest possible;
– lunch is normal, or often light;
– dinner is always too big.

The arguments which are generally used to excuse these regrettable practises are that:

– in the morning we are not hungry and have no time (we have already mentioned this;
– at lunch time work is the priority, unless you have a business lunch;
– the evening is the only time of relaxation when the family can be together and possibly sit down to a good dinner which is even more welcome as you are hungry.

When a television journalist was asked one day how she had been able to accept taking on the early morning broadcasts, which meant she had to get up at four in the morning, she replied: *"I only had to change my eating habits!"*. As I have already said, this is the only thing that I am going to ask you to do.

Thousands of people like you have already done it, and there is no reason why you yourself should not manage it. You will if you really want to. Your success will in any case be the measure of your determination.

Breakfast

As we have pointed out earlier, this must be substantial. Given that this is the first stage of what will be your newly found vitality, it must be given the necessary time
Get up quarter of an hour or twenty minutes earlier. This will be even easier as you will have slept noticeably better because you have followed all our advice, particularly that concerning the evening meal.

1. First of all, the vitamins

As many of you consume an amount of vitamins very close to the danger level, and others only vaguely remember their existence, you will have to rebuild your vitamin stocks.
It must be realised that the absence of, or at least a deficiency in vitamins is an important factor in tiredness. The Vitamin B group, and Vitamin C are particularly relevant. Some may think that getting them where they are easily found, in the chemists, will be good enough.
If necessary, you may have to, but for various reasons, only if there is no natural solution.

First of all, it is a question of principle. If we are happy to accept the idea that modern food is lacking in essential nutrients and that to re-establish the balance all you need to do is fall back on synthetic pharmaceutical products, this will not help to resolve the dramatic dilemma of our times: that the agro-food business is no longer at all concerned about the nutritional content of its products.

In the future, if the air is so polluted that it is unbreathable, it will probably be easier just to advise everyone to wear a mask or even to regularly buy doses of oxygen, as they already do in Japan.

It would, however, be easier to do away with pollution, but on the one hand that would be too "green", and on the other, many potential markets could thereby stupidly escape clever businessmen. That of course would be a pity.

Finally, whatever doses are taken, synthetic vitamins are less well assimilated than natural vitamins in a foodstuff. This is because in natural food there are substances which are not very well understood and which have the effect of improving their absorption.

To get your daily ration of vitamin B, all you have to do is eat brewer's yeast, which is a completely natural product. You can find it everywhere (in chain stores, chemists) and in specialised shops [1]. This yeast should therefore be taken as a cure for a month during the whole of PHASE I, and then every other month.

As we have already said large doses of Vitamin B should help make you less tired, but you should very quickly notice other results such as stronger nails and healthier hair. In addition, brewer's yeast contains chromium which helps to correct hyperinsulinism.

---

1. The Michel MONTIGNAC boutique, 160 Old Brompton Road, London SW5 0BA, Tel/Fax: 0171 370 2010

2. Fruit and Vitamin C

You can start your breakfast by drinking fresh fruit juice (lemon, pineapple, or even orange). You can also eat a fruit, and the kiwi fruit would be the best, because it has five times as much Vitamin C as oranges for a smaller volume.

If the fruit is freshly squeezed, it must be drunk immediately, as any delay will lead to a considerable loss of vitamins. It is silly to drink ready prepared fruit juice, even if it is so-called "pure fruit", as its vitamin content has long since nearly or completely disappeared.

It also important to note that whatever fruit is chosen for breakfast, it should be eaten before anything else, on an empty stomach.

Contrary to traditional practice, fruit should never be eaten at the end of a meal because it is a food which takes little time to digest (about fifteen minutes). When you eat a fruit, it goes into the stomach but does not remain there, as it has no job. It therefore quickly goes into the small intestine where it is digested and absorbed. If the fruit is eaten at the end of a meal it goes into the stomach after the pylorus has closed because other foods have been eaten which necessitate two to three hours digestion (meat, fish, fats).

The fruit will thus be a prisoner in a hot and wet environment which will lead to its fermentation and upset the digestive process of the other foods, at the same time losing most of its Vitamins.

This is why, apart from the fact that you have to drop the habit of eating fruit at the end of meals, it is necessary to begin with them at breakfast.

We would even recommend that you wait fifteen to twenty minutes after eating a fruit, so as so enable it to reach the small intestine and not run the risk of being locked into the stomach when other food is eaten.

117

As far as cooked fruit is concerned, this limitation will not be exactly the same, as it does not run the risk of fermenting. It seems that we can tolerate it better, especially as far as marmalade without sugar is concerned, as it contains less Vitamin C.

Various breakfast formulæ

The main aim of PHASE I is obviously to lose excess weight. But one of the other aims we are trying for is also, and above all, to give the pancreas a chance to go back to normal activity. As we saw in the previous chapters, it has been abnormally stimulated to produce insulin through over-consumption of hyperglycaemic foods.

We were able to show that a breakfast of white bread, sugar, honey or jam was the root cause of often feeling out of salts (sudden tiredness) at the end of the morning. The poor pancreas, abused for so many years, needs to more or less get its health back in order to lose this hypersensitivity which is the cause of its tendency to hyperinsulinism. We will be asking less of it then for a while, so that it can go back to its normal state. All the breakfast formulae we will be proposing will therefore take this into account.

1. Carbohydrate breakfast

This should be taken as often as possible, and especially at home. It will be totally made up of a choice of, or all of:

Good carbohydrates (glucides):
- wholemeal bread;
- whole cereals, without sugar;
- sugarless jams and marmalades.

Milk products

• *fromage blanc* (skimmed cream cheese) with 0 % fat, or low-fat yoghurt.

Drinks

• skimmed milk;
• decaffeinated coffee [2]
• weak tea
• chicory
• Soya juice.

All kind of fats (butter, margarine) and full fat milk products are excluded from this breakfast.

a. Good carbohydrates

Wholemeal bread

As we are going to advise you not to eat bread (except occasionally) for the two other meals for a balanced diet, it is preferable to eat it without restriction for breakfast.

Bread, yes, but not any old bread. First of all it must be wholemeal, that is to say that it must be made with all the components of the wheat grain. This must not be confused with such things as malted wheat bread, and various "brown" breads, which are bit ambiguous, as the flour from which they are made is not as "whole" as you might think. Sometimes they contain most of the components of the wheat grain, but some of them have been eliminated and it is difficult to know in what proportion.

You might think that various "grain" breads have been made entirely with whole flour, but usually they are made with white flour with added grain. This is either to make

---

2. We are, of course referring to real and not instant coffee.

it look better or to make it easier to manufacture. It is not always easy to find real wholemeal bread made entirely of whole wheat grains.

Likewise, bran bread, it is only white bread to which the baker has added bran [3].

What proportions are necessary? This is the problem, as bakers have a tendency not to add much bran. This is not because it is expensive, but the mixture then becomes much more difficult to knead. A bran bread with less than 20 % bran could be alright, but even though it may have enough fibre to lower glycaemia, it will still be lacking in the totality of the necessary vitamins and mineral salts.

If you do not find real whole bread at your baker's this would not be surprising as it is still infrequent, and the best thing to do would be to buy it by mail order. It is sold toasted and dried, and will keep for several months. It is cheaper than the average bread and even more competitive as it is made with yeast and organic flours [4].

What are you going to put on your wholemeal bread?

There are several possible options according to taste. You can use *fromage blanc* with 0 % fat, or marmalade without sugar, or even both together.

Jams and marmalades without sugar have nothing to do with low sugar jams, which you must be careful of, as in the best cases, they only have 10 – 15 % less sugar. That means that instead of 55 % sugar they only have 45 %.

Without sugar they contain 100 % fruit (cooked naturally in its juice), 0 % sugar and pectin (soluble fibre). You can also buy them by mail order or in specialised shops.

You should be warned that if you chose the *fromage blanc*

---

3. It must be emphasised here that the bran *must* be of organic origin, and this is rarely the case at the bakers. Normal bran is in fact a concentrate of pesticides, insecticides and herbicides.

4. MONTIGNAC products, including toasted dried bread, can be obtained from the Michel MONTIGNAC Boutique in London (see address previous pages).

option (with or without jam or marmalade), it is important that this should be 0 % fat).

Cereals

In everyday speech the word cereal usually refers to breakfast cereals, especially those for children, which are made of maize flakes, corn flakes or puffed rice.

If you should have forgotten their noble American pedigree, I would remind you that these products are full of sugar, covered in caramel or have added honey and chocolate, all of which have to be excluded during this phase of slimming.

The cereals we recommend, which come in flake form, are of course whole cereals, from organic sources. They have no added sugar etc.

Meuslis, which contain walnuts, hazelnuts, almonds and dry fruit, can be good too, if you only need to lose a few pounds. For those who need to lose more (more than 20 kilos), it would be better to wait until PHASE II to give yourself a chance of losing them as quickly as possible.

Flake cereals and meusli can be mixed with *fromage blanc* with 0 % fat or with yoghurt or even hot or cold milk (skimmed of course).

These cereals should be chewed slowly and well moistened with saliva in order to be easily digestible. Ideally, you should grind them yourself with a suitable machine. The maximum amount of Vitamins are obtained when grain is freshly ground or milled.

A breakfast of fruit is equally possible, if for example you are on holiday in an exotic location. But do at least add a skimmed milk product in order to have a high enough input of proteins and calcium.

b. Drinks

Just as you have to eat breakfast, you must also drink a lot. The body needs maximum rehydration when you awake.

Coffee

As far as coffee is concerned, it would be preferable to get out of the caffeine habit (at least in PHASE I), as for some susceptible people it has the effect of stimulating insulin secretion when the pancreas is in bad condition. Some authors do however attribute the property of helping to melt fat to it.

Much has been said about coffee and sometimes contradictory things. Let's take this opportunity to say something about some aspects of coffee.

It is true that in the past, the industrial decaffeination process was more toxic than the caffeine. This is no longer the case. Decaffeinated coffee may be taken, within reason, especially as it has now become very good, at least in France, where decaffeinated ground coffee can now be found in the cafés. We can recommend either decaffeinated or, and this would be much better, a mixture of decaffeinated coffee and chicory. If you like coffee with milk and have no problem with this, there is no reason to go without.

The idea that milk is a poison is without foundation, which does not mean that some people should nevertheless avoid it. It is all a question of individual sensitivity. Sometimes it is an enzyme deficiency that prevents some people from digesting milk, and in addition, the coffee/milk mixture may be worse as coffee changes the structure of milk.

Tea

Although tea contains a bit of caffeine, it can be taken as it stands, as long as it is not too strong.

Tea has interesting diuretic properties and some Asians also affirm that certain Chinese teas help slim, but this has not been scientifically proved.

Milk

Skimmed milk is preferable, as whole milk is not very digestible for an adult, and in addition is too rich in bad saturated fats.

Powder milk would be best, as you can get a thicker milk when less water is added.

c. Artificial sweeteners

It is obvious that white refined sugar must be forever banished, and especially for breakfast.

But behind sugar there lurks the taste of sugar, and it is precisely this that you must gradually lose the habit of.

You therefore have, if not to get off it entirely, at least become less accustomed to it by getting used to having less. Someone once said: *"Sugar is what gives a bad taste to coffee when there isn't one"*.

However, all those who have given up sugar in their coffee would not go back to it again for all the world.

To lower your sugar consumption you will be able to substitute artificial sweeteners.

Much as been said about artificial sweeteners and controversy still rages on this subject.

The financial implications for these products are immense, and their detractors (sugar manufacturers) as well as advocates (the pharmaceutical companies that manufacture them) have been competing with studies on their bad effects or lack of effects; they seem to have more or less come out of this unscathed.

Even though they may not be toxic, nothing proves that they may not be so when consumed for long periods over many years. This is the same problem that we have with all chemical food additives. Who can say what their long-term effects will be on the body?

We would therefore recommend that (if necessary) they should be used very sparingly. They should only be taken to get past the transition stage and progressively be, if not abandoned, at least only used at very long intervals.

Recent French and American studies have tended to show that even if some sweeteners are not themselves toxic, they do have a tendency to destabilise the metabolism in the long term by upsetting the glycaemic level for the following meal.

When taken during a meal sweeteners do not modify glycaemia and lead to no risk of insulin secretion. However, if the next meal contains carbohydrates, the glycaemic curve runs the risk of abnormal increase, even when the carbohydrate has a low glycaemic index.

The risk in PHASE I would be rather limited, as the meals are either protein-lipid (fat), or protein-glucide (carbohydrate).

The danger might be greater in PHASE II, but we will come back to this later. This gives you another reason to take advantage of PHASE I to get over your sweet tooth. As for fructose, the merits of which have been praised, both because it does not cause cancer and because its glycaemic index is low, it is mainly recommended for making deserts. It has, however, been accused of encouraging increase in triglyceride level. In reality, this is only the case for those for whom this is a serious problem and only when they go over 100 grams a day, which is a huge quantity.

If you follow the principles of the method (as we will see below), it will lead to a very substantial lowering of triglycerides, and fructose may be used sparingly to make pastries.

2. Savoury protein-lipid breakfast

Another variation for breakfast would be the formula consisting of eating meat, pork products (bacon, ham, sausages, eggs, cheese, etc. This is more or less the Anglo-Saxon breakfast with one important difference: carbohy-

124

Carbohydrate breakfast

RECOMMENDED	TOLERATED	FORBIDDEN
Fresh fruit juice A fruit (eaten 15 min before) Wholemeal bread Raw cereals without sugar Unsweetened marmalade 0 % fat *fromage blanc* 0 % fat yoghurt Powdered skimmed milk Decaffeinated coffee Chicory	Wholemeal bread Bran bread White bread Meusli High fibre crispbread German black bread Wholemeal Swedish crispbread Unsweetened Cooked fruit Fresh skimmed milk Tea Coffee + chicory	White bread *Biscottes* (toasted dehydrated bread) Croissant Brioche Milk roll Chocolate roll *Madeleines* (sponge type cakes Jam Honey Whole *fromage blanc* Whole or semi-skimmed milk Ordinary coffee Chocolate drink

Protein-lipid breakfast

RECOMMENDED	TOLERATED	FORBIDDEN
Scrambled eggs Hard boiled eggs Fried eggs Omelette Bacon Sausages (chipolatas) Cooked ham White ham Cheeses Skimmed milk or semi-skimmed Decaffeinated coffee Chicory	Fruit juice (drunk 1/4 hour before Whole milk Coffee + chicory Tea	White bread Wholemeal bread *Biscottes* Croissant Milk roll Chocolate roll *Madeleine* Jam Honey Cereals Ordinary coffee Chocolate drink Fruit

drates are totally excluded, and that goes for good carbo-hydrates too (no bread).

Another reservation: as this breakfast includes a notable

quantity of saturated fats, it is imperative that those suffering from hypercholesterolemia exclude it.

If you do adopt it, it is better to have a dinner without lipids (fats), built around good carbohydrates, and to have fruit at tea time.

This is in fact the kind of breakfast that you can get most readily in hotels, as the traditional morning buffet generally has a wide selection of possibilities. As far as drinks are concerned, the recommendations made for the carbohydrate formula breakfast should be applied.

A skimmed milk product must be added to this kind of breakfast (milk, *fromage blanc*, yoghurt).

Snacks

If you are used to munching something during the morning, it is probably because you are a little hypoglycaemic. By following the recommendations in this chapter, which will especially lead you to adopt a less hyperglycaemic

All Fruit Breakfast

RECOMMENDED	TOLERATED	FORBIDDEN
Orange Mandarin Grapefruit Kiwi Apple Pear Mango Strawberries Blackberries Figs Apricot Nectarine Plum	Grapes Cherries Hazelnuts Prunes Dates Dry fruit	Banana Preserved Fruit salad Crystallised fruit

126

breakfast, you should soon be able to lose the need to put something in your stomach around eleven o'clock.

If, however, you should still want to eat something during your coffee break, and this may be a habit at work, take advantage of this to eat a fruit, an apple for example, unless you would prefer to eat a few almonds, walnuts or hazelnuts (which are very rich in Vitamin C), or even some wholemeal bread.

You may also have a piece of cheese (low-fat if possible). You can now find small individual portions of cheese that can easily be carried around without giving off an unwelcome smell. A hard-boiled egg would also be acceptable.

Lunch

Lunch should also respect one of the fundamental aims set in this PHASE I, which is to not make much demand on the pancreas.

As for breakfast, its quantity is not limited. If must however be big enough to make you feel full.

It will also include generally:

– a starter;
– a main dish with a very good carbohydrate (with a very low glycaemic index, as for example in green vegetables);
– cheese or yoghurt.

It must be eaten without bread.

1. The starter

This can consist of *crudités* (raw vegetables), meat, fish, eggs, seafood or crustaceans.

a. Crudités (raw vegetables)

This is far and away the starter that you should always prefer. Raw vegetables generally include a large amount of fibres, and these fill the stomach well.

They also contain mineral salts and vitamins, which will be all the better assimilated when the vegetables are not cooked. Amongst them we can recommend:

- tomatoes;
- cucumbers;
- celery;
- mushrooms;
- green beans
- leeks;
- palm hearts;
- cabbage (red or white)
- cauliflower;
- avocado;
- broccoli;
- artichokes;
- gherkins
- radishes.

And also all the green salad vegetables:

- lettuce;
- chicory;
- lamb's lettuce;
- dandelion leaves;
- endive lettuce;
- watercress.

The *crudités* can be seasoned with a normal dressing of wine vinegar, oil, salt and pepper and possibly mustard.

As far as possible, priority should be given to olive oil, which ensures good prevention against cardio-vascular diseases.

Celery can be grated and mixed with mayonnaise *(rémou-*

128

lade). In like manner, cucumber can be dressed either with a little low fat *crème fraiche* or preferably with 0 % fat *fromage blanc*.

Naturally, ready made mayonnaise and salad dressings should be completely outlawed, as they contain sugar and other undesirable additives, like starch and various suspect flours.

Among possible raw vegetables that are often available in restaurants and canteens and that should be forgotten during PHASE I are the following:

- carrots;
- potatoes;
- maize;
- rice;
- pearl barley
- lentils (which come back in PHASE II)
- dried beans (which come back in PHASE II).

You may have walnuts, hazelnuts and pinenuts in your salads, though you must absolutely not have any croutons.

b. Fish

Jump at the opportunity to have fish whenever you can. You will have already understood that the more fatty the fish (sardines, herrings, mackerel, wild salmon), the better it contributes to lowering cholesterol, triglycerides and the protection of your arteries.

Do not therefore hesitate to eat salmon, especially marinated in olive oil *(carpaccio)*. When you are in a restaurant it is the ideal starter.

I would remind you though that most fish or crustaceans can also be had as starters:

- sardines (grilled or with olive oil if possible);
- mackerel;
- herrings (though not with the undesirable potatoes of course);

129

– anchovies;
– tuna;
– shrimps;
– scallops;
– gambas and scampi;
– lobsters and crayfish
– crab;
– caviar and its substitutes;
– all other shellfish.

Langoustines and oysters which contain some carbohydrates should be avoided during **PHASE I**, especially if you need to lose a lot of weight. They will come back in **PHASE II** with no limitations.

It is obvious that all the fish pastes and pâtés will be welcome, as long as they have been "home made", or rather as long as they have not been industrially manufactured, as is unfortunately more and more often the case.

When they are made in the industrial food industry circuit, these ready made pâtés are full of additives: binding agents based on flour, or starch, sugar in all its forms (glucose syrup and other polydextroses) and the unavoidable sodium glutamate which gives it its great "more-ish" taste.

Get into the habit of nagging your suppliers into giving you the composition of their products. The more they realise the problem, the more they will have to take notice of it.

c. Pork products

The first thing to observe concerning pork products is that you must go slowly and be a bit wary about them. Firstly because they contain high quantities of saturated fats (which vary according to the part of the pig and the way it has been treated). Then, because when such products are marketed through the distribution circuits they are stuffed with additives (nitrates). But, and above all, because they are made with doubtful quality meat; usually pork from concentration camp type of farming.

130

Limit your intake and always check the quality.

A few years ago, traditional French families who had not completely cut off from their roots and rural origin still used to "fatten a pig". Usually they went halves with a peasant. They bought two small sucking pigs and gave them to a farmer. The latter fed them traditionally and when they grew up, one of them came back to you. All that you had to do then was "cook the pig".

In all French villages, if you ask the local policeman or the priest (if there is still one) they will give you the address of a team of specialists who will come to your the house or the country house of your friends to cook your pig and make you blood sausages, pâtés, joints, cutlets and hams, ready usually to be put in the freezer of your town flat.

This will of course be cheaper than if you had bought them in the supermarket, but above all they will be incontestably better from every point of view, especially for your health and that of your family. But these "pig parties" are above all a unique opportunity of renewed contact with nature a salutary return to your roots.

d. Eggs

When eggs are fresh and come from a traditional farm, their yellow is a little copper coloured. They then are of exceptional nutritional value, as they contain many vitamins (A, D, K, E, B8, B9 and B12, in quantities which are of course related to their quality.

Eggs do of course contain saturated fats, but the are not readily assimilated because of the presence of lecithin.

Risk of cardio-vascular disease will therefore be less if you should have hypercholesterolemia. Eggs can be used for many starters: hard-boiled, egg mayonnaise, omelette, fried eggs, etc.

e. Other possible starters

According to circumstances and everyone's imagination, or at least that of the Chef, many foods in the categories mentioned above can be happily mixed together, as in a *salade niçoise* or *assiette landaise* (mixed platter of sliced salamis and pork products)

When eating out in a restaurant if you order a starter including a variety of foods, make sure you ask the waiter or the *maître d'hôtel* what exactly is in it. If you are not careful to check, you may find yourself with carrots, rice, maize or croutons mixed in with the rest.

Be especially careful when you order a salad with bacon *(salade aux lardons)* as the bacon is shrinking to the advantage of the undesirable croutons.

Among other possible starters, we would mention cheese, which is often a heated goats cheese (Chavignol) on a bed of green salad. There again, insist that it should be served without toast.

As for *foie gras,* we have left it out of our list, as it is quite exceptional. Although it has nutritional virtues which are still not well understood, we would treat it with a little reservation as far as eating it during PHASE I is concerned. It in fact contains a high proportion of mono-unsaturated fat (oleic acid) which has the property of protecting the cardio-vascular system.

Foie gras is in fact a mixture of carbohydrates (glycogen) and lipids. This is why it is not recommended in PHASE I, at least for those who have a lot of weight to lose.

Toast which is usually served with it is forbidden anyway in PHASE I.

f. Forbidden starters

Some may think that everything that is not authorised is forbidden.

This is an error! There is such a wide variety of products that our lists will never be exhaustive. Inasmuch as you know the basic rules of our approach, it will be easy for you to determine if any food (something exotic, for example) which is not on the list is acceptable or not. Then, in most cases, you only have to reason by analogy.

132

The same goes for all that has to be excluded from your food. At the point where you are, you are easily able to make a judgement when you see something different on a menu or on your plate.

Nevertheless, here is a list of most of them:

 – vol au vents and other flaky pastry dishes;
 – quiches or pies;
 – soufflés made with white flour;
 – white pasta;
 – white rice (especially non-stick);
 – refined semolina;
 – anything made with potatoes.

2. The main course

The main course for lunch should always be made up of meat, poultry or fish accompanied by the vegetables that are on the list of very good carbohydrates, that is, those with a glycaemic index below 15. These will therefore mostly be green vegetables which have a high fibre content.

a. Meat

Apart from the fact that it is best to eat fish if you have a choice, if you do not have meat, you should choose from amongst the meat dishes those which have the least fat, so that you can limit as far as possible your consumption of saturated fats.

Beef, lamb, mutton and pork are rather fatty meats (veal less so). Poultry is therefore better on this level. Even *magret de canard* (sliced red duck meat) has a much lower level of saturated fats and a high level of unsaturated fats (the good ones) that only poultry can boast of.

Of course, you must be careful of stews and casseroles which, in many cases will be served swimming in gravy "cemented" with white flour, but this is luckily something you will not find in the best restaurants.

Be careful too of veal cutlets which are often breaded, rolled in bread crumbs which are undesirable according to our principles.

b. Fish

All fish, without exception, may be chosen, the only reservation being that they should not be cooked in bread crumbs or rolled in flour before being fried.   As always, if you are in a restaurant, ask about the way it has been cooked.   Only accept fish which has been boiled or grilled.

Dressings should be regarded with the same caution as meat.   The best of them will always be a mixture of lemon juice and virgin olive oil, which is very rich in vitamins, as you know.

At home, frozen fish is the best guarantee of freshness. Buy hake or cod fillets and cook them as they are, either in a simplified stock of mixed herbs *(herbes de Provence)* using one soup spoon for a litre of water, or on a very low setting in a covered frying pan in which you have put just a few drops of olive oil.

c. Side dishes

Before ordering a dish in a restaurant, and this should become second nature, you should instinctively ask the eternal question: *"what does it come with"*

Nine times out of ten the waiter will answer, certain of pleasing you: *"chips, or fried potatoes"*.   If you ask for something else, he will invariably reply: *"rice or else pasta"*.

In these cases I have often been tempted to dash into the kitchen to throw all the Chef's saucepans and bad carbohydrates at his head, to punish him for so little creativity.

If I have never done so, it is not so much because I am "well brought up" but rather because I know that the poor thing is not responsible.   They tell me sadly: *"why do any-*

134

thing else when 80 % of the customers refuse anything but the ubiquitous potatoes, pasta and rice".

Some Chefs, amongst the greatest, even manage, just like the worst of our school cooks, to tempt us into their sanctuaries after weeks of waiting, just to concoct some kind of old fashioned mashed potato dish. They still manage keep the admiration of the best gastronomic guides.

How can a "star" of cooking be so lacking in judgement when they are by definition exceptionally creative?

We cannot be too hard on the local fast food outlet, or orphanage canteen if they have not "thrown away the spuds", but when potatoes can be found in the middle of the best gastronomic menus, in a country which fattened its pigs for centuries, this seems really making fun of us, especially when they are charged at the same rate as truffles.

Examples of lack of coherence in food **choices** like this are not lacking. When you go to Guadeloupe for the first time, you expect to be served a very special selection of exotic vegetables that all the botany books mention. In fact, nothing of the sort. This dream island which could be a real oasis and export its special tropical vegetables to the whole world, produces nothing. Their food is made up of white rice and potatoes, which are of course imported.

I myself had more difficulty in Pointe-à-Pitre than in Paris in finding a restaurant which could serve up a good mashed Christophines, a local food which is really different.

In the same way, we may be astonished to find that Creole rice can be so much the symbol of local cooking in that country, when it has never been produced there but was imposed by the Indians who came to replace the black slaves at the time of emancipation.

Therefore, when you are eating in a restaurant, make sure that you get something different from what others are having. If you insist a bit you will even be surprised to see that it is always possible to have green beans, spinach, cauliflower or even broccoli.

If you really cannot get any of these, make do with a salad and shame your host.

The vegetables that we can recommend in PHASE I are the following:

- courgettes;
- aubergines;
- tomatoes;
- broccoli
- spinach;
- turnips
- swedes;
- parsnips;
- Jerusalem artichokes
- peppers;
- fennel;
- celery;
- sorel
- green beans;
- bettes
- mushrooms;
- salsify
- cabbage
- cauliflower;
- sauerkraut;
- Brussels sprouts.

But this list is certainly not exhaustive.

3. Cheese or desert?

In PHASE I you will most often have to make do with cheese. You are going to object that it will be difficult to eat your cheese without bread or biscuits. In fact it is just as easy as not putting sugar in your coffee. When you manage it, you wonder how you did otherwise for so long.

One trick to enable you to get there without transition is that of eating the cheese with the salad.

Another possibility as a replacement for the plinth that bread constitutes for the cheese is to use a piece of hard cheese (Dutch for example) to eat a soft cheese (*fromage frais*).

For all those, including the women, who really want to lose weight, they should know that it is not recommended to eat large quantities of *fromage blanc* and *fromage frais* even when it is 0 % fat.

It contains quite a bit of carbohydrates (galactose) in the liquid and if you eat a lot you could find at the end of the meal that your secretion of insulin has gone up again with the risk of storing the fats which were eaten previously.

A ration of 80 to 100 grams should be a maximum. As far as possible, you must always chose *fromage blanc* which has been strained and avoid those which have been whipped.

As for deserts, except occasionally, you should cut them out during PHASE I, as it is unlikely that you will find any without sugar, or even without fructose. At home you can always make *œufs à la neige* (whipped eggs) or eggs in milk, if necessary adding an artificial sweetener, but be careful of what we said about that earlier.

The Quick Snack Lunch

Perhaps for various reasons you may not have the time to lunch properly.

Before this, you managed with a sandwich, but now, at least in PHASE I, this is completely outlawed. You will see that you may possibly eat them again, occasionally, in PHASE II, on condition that they are made with wholemeal bread.

As we have explained, it is important never to miss a meal and we shall therefore have to find at least a minimum way of feeding you at lunch time! Several solutions can be proposed:

1. Eat fruit

Any fruit meal is acceptable, except for bananas which are too high in carbohydrates (glycaemic index of 60).

Eat three or four apples for example, or alternate them with oranges.

Eat two apples with 200 grams of walnuts, hazelnuts or almonds (they can all be found ready shelled), and you can complement these with two yoghurts.

2. Eat cheese

Any cheese will do as long as it is has as little fat as possible (otherwise you will soon be tired of it) and does not smell too strongly if you should, for example, be eating it in your office.

A small carton of 250 grams of 0 % fat *fromage blanc* with a few added raspberries, strawberries or kiwis might make a change from time to time.

These are in fact about the only fruit, together perhaps with blackberries, which do not keep to the rule we set that fruit should be eaten on an empty stomach.

These fruits run very little risk of fermenting in the stomach. If you eat them with 0 % fat *fromage frais* it won't be the end of the world. We will see later that they are even acceptable at the end of a normal meal in PHASE II.

You could even eat two or three hard-boiled eggs. If you eat them with pieces of raw tomato and no dressing they seem less filling

3. Bread

Doing without bread for the two main meals (especially if they contain fat) is one of the basic principles that it is important to respect. Maybe you think that we could have been less dogmatic and only forbidden white bread.

Maybe. But will you find wholemeal bread in the restaurants you go to? There is usually little chance of finding any in restaurants.

Then, even if it is wholemeal, bread is unnecessary with a big meal. It has the drawback of blowing up the stomach, making you feel heavy and can contribute to an increase in the well-known feeling of sleepiness after a meal.

And then, in PHASE I the aim is to stimulate the pancreas as little as possible. In a protein-lipid meal, the least secretion of insulin, even if it is not enough to build reserve fats, could put a brake on weight loss. You will not get fatter but you will not get slimmer either.

4. Wine

Like bread, during PHASE I of weight loss, you are advised to do without wine altogether, above all if you need to lose a lot of weight.

If your weight is not too great, you could just have half a glass at the end of the meal, particularly with cheese.

In PHASE II we will come back to this and the way in which it should be drunk and also talk about the bad habits that you have to lose.

It would be better only to drink water during PHASE I, or even tea. Many English people do drink tea with their meals and enjoy it, as well as seeing its beneficial effects. Tea actually has the digestive properties that can be attributed to all hot drinks. This is why, if you prefer them, you should not hesitate to drink herbal teas (without sugar) with

139

your meals. None of them have any bad effects – on the contrary, they are all beneficial.

Dinner

As we have already mentioned, dinner should be the lightest meal of the day. Unfortunately, for social, or professional reasons, it is often the excuse for a veritable feast, either at home or elsewhere (an outing, at a friend's house).

It is easy to change your habits at home. As breakfast is now more substantial and you now have lunch, dinner does not need to be as copious as it used to be.

The same reasoning can be applied to dinner as to lunch as far as its composition is concerned, but taking care to limit fat quantities and avoid meat if you already had some at lunch time.

When eating at home you should, as far as possible, try to begin with a good old-fashioned home made vegetable soup: leeks, celery, turnips, cabbage (no potatoes!), and then eat a small omelette with green salad.

But dinner should above all be the time to go back to lost traditions, rehabilitating some pulses that nowadays are rarely eaten, like lentils, beans and peas.

It is a good idea to be able to have two or three protein-carbohydrate dinners a week, which means they should be made up mostly of carbohydrates with a low or very low glyceamic index. The only rule that must be kept in PHASE I is that these dinners absolutely must be cooked and eaten without fat.

You could start, for example, with a good vegetable soup (without potatoes or carrots) or creamed mushroom or tomato soup, with no fat of course.

Lentils, beans and peas can be mixed with some onion,

sieved tomato (*coulis de tomate)* or a mushroom sauce (see annexes).

Wholemeal pasta is another possibility, together with brown rice or whole semolina[6] and these can be made more interesting by serving them with vegetables and a non-fat sauce or *coulis*. These foods also have the added benefit of containing vegetable proteins, fibres, B vitamins and many mineral salts.

Desert after a carbohydrate dinner can only be 0 % fat *fromage blanc*, yoghurt (possibly seasoned with sugarless jam or marmalade) or cooked fruit. You could possibly eat a little wholemeal bread with this kind of meal, but it might be a bit too filling.

As for lunch, the recommended drinks for dinner in PHASE I are water, weak tea or herbal teas. Occasionally you may have a small glass of red wine.

If you had a big meal at lunch time (for example, a business lunch) and you want to eat lightly in the evening, there again, you can eat only fruit and a yoghurt, or some cereal and a skimmed milk product.

---

6. These products can be obtained from the Montignac Boutique in London, 160 Old Brompton Road, London SW5 0BA, Tel/Fax 0171 370 2010.

Protein-lipid meal, PHASE I
With very low glycaemic index carbohydrates

STARTERS			
RAW VEGETABLES	**FISH**	**PORK PRODUCTS**	**OTHERS**

RECOMMENDED
Asparagus
Tomatoes
Cucumbers
Artichokes
Peppers
Celery
Mushrooms
Green beans
Leeks
Palm hearts
Cabbage
Cauliflower
Gherkins
Avocado
Bean sprouts
Lettuce
Chicory salad
Lamb's lettuce
Dandelion
Chicory lettuce
Water cress
Broccoli
Radishes
	Smoked salmon
	Marinated salmon
	Sardines
	Mackerel
	Herrings
	Anchovies
	Tun
	Cod liver
	Shrimps
	Scallops
	Gambas
	Langoustine
	Lobster
	Caviar
	Cockles
	Clams
	Winkles
	Crab
	Whelks
	Calamaris
	Octopus
	Oysters
		Salamis
		Uncooked ham
		White ham
		Chipolata
		Dried sausage
		Muzzle (*museau*)
		Head in aspic
		  (*fromage de*
		  tête)
		Dried beef
		  (*grison*)
		Salad with bacon
		  (*frisée*
		  aux lardons)
		Salad with giz-
		zards
		  (*salade*
		  de gésiers)
		Rillettes
		Pâtés
			Mozzarella
			Hot goat's cheese
			Veal sweetbreads
			Frog legs
			Snails
			Omelette
			Hard boiled eggs
			Scrambles eggs
			Egg Benedict
			Eggs in aspic
			Fish soup

FORBIDDEN	**TO AVOID**	**TO AVOID**	**TO BANNISH**
Carrots Beet Maize Rice Semolina Lentils Dried beans Potatoes	Langoustines Oysters	*Foie gras* *Boudin blanc* (Chitterlings) Terrines contain- ing flour	Puff pastry Vol-au-vent Quiche Pancakes Soufflés Blinis Toast Croutons Pizza Deep fried batter Cheese fondue

142

Protein-lipid meal, PHASE I
With very low glycaemic index carbohydrates

	MAIN DISH			
	FISH	MEAT	POULTRY	PORK, OFFAM, GAME

RECOMMENDED	Salmon
	Mackerel
	Tuna
	Sardines
	Herrings
	Perch
	Cod
	Plaice
	Sole
	Lemon sole
	Monkfish
	Whiting
	Cod
	Red mullet
	Trout
	And generally all
	  sea and fresh
	  water fish
		Beef
		Veal
		Pork
		Mutton
		Lamb
			Chicken
			Hen
			Capon
			Guinea fowl
			Turkey
			Goose
			Duck
			Quail
			Pheasant
			Pigeon
			Rabbit
				Hare
				Wild rabbit
				Venison
				Boar
				Chitterlings
				Black pudding
				Ham
				Beef heart
				Beef tongue
				Veal sweetbreads
				Kidneys
				Pigs trotters

	TO BANNISH	TO AVOID	TO AVOID	TO AVOID
	Breaded fish	Fatty parts	Skin	Liver

143

Protein-lipid meal, PHASE I
With very low glycaemic index carbohydrates

SIDE DISHES	
RECOMMENDED	TO BANNISH
Green beans	Couscous
Broccoli	Lentils
Aubergine	Dried beans
Courgette	Peas
Spinach	Chestnuts
Mushrooms	Potatoes
Salsifis	Carrots
Celery	Rice
Bettes	Pasta
Sorrel	
Turnips	
Leeks	
Tomatoes	
Onions	
Peppers	
Ratatouille	
Cauliflower	
Cabbage	
Sauerkraut	
Christophine	
Green salads	
Vegetable mousse (pâté without potatoes)	
Artichokes	

Protein-carbohydrate meal, PHASE I
fibre rich

	STARTERS	MAIN COURSE	DESSERT

Good carbohydrates to choose from	Vegetable soup
	Cream
	  of mushroom
	  soup
	
	Pumpkin soup
	Cream of tomato
	  soup
		Lentils
		Dried beans
		Peas
		Broad beans
		Brown rice
		Wholemeal pasta
		Wholemeal
		  semolina
			0 % fat *fromage blanc*
			0 % fat yoghurt
			Fruit compote
			Cooked fruit
			Unsweetened Jam
			  or marmalade

Recommended	Without fat,
	  potatoes
	  or carrots
		Without fat, served with tomato *coulis* or mushroom sauce [7] or with a vegetable side dish	Without fats or sugar

Condiments, ingredients, seasonings
and various spices

TO EAT:				TO BANNISH
WITHOUT RESTRICTION			IN REASONABLE QUANTITY	

Gherkins
Pickles
Small onions
Home-made
French-
  dressing
Nuoc-mam
Green olives
Black olives
Tapenade
Celery salt
	Oils:
	Olive
	Sunflower
	Groundnut
	Walnut
	Hazelnut
	Grapeseed
	
	Lemon
	Parmesan
	Gruyère
		Parsley
		Tarragon
		Garlic
		Onion
		Shallots
		Thyme
		Bay leaf
		Cinnamon
		Basilica
		Chives
		Savoury
		Fennel
			Mustard
			Salt
			Pepper
			Mayonnaise
			Béarnaise
			  sauce
			Hollandaise
			  sauce
			Fresh cream
			  sauce
				Potato starch
				Cornflour
				Tomato
				  ketchup
				Bought
				  mayonnaise
				White sauce
				Flour-based
				  sauce
				Sugar
				Caramel
				Palm oil
				Paraffin oil

---

7. See recipes in Annexes.

Special advice

1. Be careful of sauces

Traditional sauces and other dressings are often made from white flour. You should henceforth avoid them like the plague.

More modern sauces (*nouvelle cuisine*) are usually made by stirring a little, usually lower fat, cream into the cooking dish. The same result will be obtained using 0 % fat *fromage blanc*.

To make a sauce that will go well with a white meat, you only have to mix some low-fat fresh cream or 0 % fat *fromage blanc* with a seasoned mustard, slightly heat it, and serve it on the meat. If you add some button mushrooms to this you won't go far wrong.

Should you wish to make a good thick sauce without flour, there is a solution: mushrooms. But for this you will need a blender. All you have to do is to completely blend the mushrooms and add the cooking liquid. This is the best way of making a tasty, smooth sauce to go with a rabbit stew or jugged hare or even with a *coq au vin* (chicken in wine).

2. Have faith in mushrooms

Button mushrooms are exceptional from every point of view, as they are an excellent fibre source and also contain many vitamins.

It is regrettable that in France they are not used as much in cooking as they are abroad.

Apart from salads, in which they can be eaten raw, they can be eaten as a dish in themselves or, at least as a side dish that generally everyone will like.

After blanching the raw mushrooms in boiling water, let

them drain for fifteen minutes. Then cut them into strips and fry them slowly in a little olive oil, add some garlic and parsley at the last minute and serve.

3. Some tips on keeping food

Those who come from a rural background may remember their mother or grandmother picking lettuce from the garden a few minutes before sitting down to a meal. The same was done for beans, tomatoes and fresh vegetables in general. At that time it was thought that vegetables, like fruit, were better picked at the last minute.

The tradition, and above all the instincts of our forefathers thereby led them, without really knowing it, to limit vitamin loss from their food, as this is linked to the time that food is kept.

Nowadays, food not only contains less vitamins at the outset than it used to, because of industrial farming methods, but the time lapse between picking and eating has considerably increased.

Spinach from intensive farming, that means methods where the output per acre is high, contained between 40 to 50 mg of vitamin C per 100 grams produced. After only one day's travel it has already lost 50 % of its vitamin content, that is about 25 mg. If it is kept two days in a refrigerator, one third of the remaining vitamin C will again be lost. There will therefore only be 16 mg remaining. If it is cooked in water, it will lose another 50 % of that.

At best, there will only remain some 8 mg of vitamin C when it gets to your plate.

If, on the other hand you are lucky enough to have a vegetable garden and you lovingly grow your spinach, as did your grandparents, the 100 grams you pick will contain at least 70 mg of vitamin C. If this is eaten the same day, you will still have 35 mg of vitamin C, that means to say about four times more than in the previous case.

147

Loss of vitamins for lettuce is even more impressive. In less than fifteen minutes it already loses 30 % of its vitamins and 48 % within the hour. We may well be shocked to learn that when lettuce finally gets onto our plates it already has a long life behind it (two to five days), and it goes without saying that salads sold ready prepared in plastic bags not only no longer contains any vitamins, but very often generously at best replace them with a dose of chemicals and at worst with salmonella.

Many restaurants boast of their fish and crustaceans which are fished live out of a tank in front of the customer minutes before serving. Why can't the same be done for lettuce?

According to specialists a cauliflower loses 2 % of its vitamins every hour. If it has been cut up, it loses 8 % every fifteen minutes, and 18 % every hour. The kitchen knife is therefore a redoubtable instrument, but nothing like the grater, which is shows no pity. Red cabbage for example may lose 62 % of its vitamin C in two hours.

The grater is in fact a veritable torture instrument for vegetables, as it multiplies by 200 the surface of the vegetable that is exposed. Red cabbage, celery and radishes undergo HSD (High Speed De-vitaminisation).

We may therefore shudder to think of the state of the vitamins in ready prepared dishes from the delicatessen counter, let alone the wrapped packaged foods we now find on the shelves of every little supermarket.

The same goes for the vegetables that are carefully chopped and grated (the day before, or even the day before that) in school, works and hospital canteens. One journalist said ironically *"You wonder what the police are up to..."* when he realised this.

4. Give thought to your cooking methods

Cooking is also the enemy of vitamins. But contrary to what you might think, it is more a question of the cooking

148

time than of cooking temperature. Blanching (at around 65 % C) destroys 90 % of the vitamin C in spinach, whereas it only loses 18 % at a temperature of 95°C. This is why a cooked food keeps better than a raw food.

The explanation is simple: enzymes (which are always greedy), which love vitamins and whose role is to destroy any product which is no longer alive (therefore as soon as it is picked), are particularly active between 50 and 65°C, whereas they are more or less neutralised at 95°C. This is why a cooked food keeps better than a raw food.

Thus, according to studies which have been done, notably by the Germans, vegetables may lose more vitamins (C, B, B2) when braised than when steamed. The shorter the cooking time, the less loss there will be. This is why it would be better to use a pressure cooker than to let them cook slowly on a low setting, as sometimes our nostalgia for the past may lead us to do. Progress has its good sides.

When cooking in water, you should however understand that most of the vitamins and mineral salts are dissolved in the cooking water. If the vegetables are organic, it is important not to throw this away, keep it to make soup, for example. If they are not organic, you may well hesitate, as in addition to the nutritional elements which we want, the cooking water contains all the pollution that we have already mentioned (nitrates, insecticides, pesticides, heavy metals, etc.).

In addition, when a vegetable fat is cooked in a frying pan, if it goes above 170° (i.e. when you cook a steak), the oil becomes saturated and is transformed into a fat which is as bad as that of meat, and this could have a bad effect on cholesterol level. Also, grilling on a barbecue has been strongly criticised in the last few years by cancer specialists.

They have noted that the burnt fats are transformed into benzopyrene, which is a substance with a high cancer risk. This is why it is more than advisable to cook meat on a vertical grill, so that the fat runs off and has no contact with the heat source.

149

As regards microwaves, since their recent introduction on the domestic market, they have been the subject of much discussion. No-one is against their highly practical side, which answers a need to economise time in today's world. But what is the real effect on the "life" of the food cooked in them? At the moment, we do not really know, as the studies which have been done are both lacking in precision and contradictory.

When you know the basic principle of a microwave oven, and most users do not, questions arise concerning what happens to vitamins, especially when you know how sensitive they are.

Food is cooked in a microwave by the heat produced by the friction of its water molecules, and this heat is transmitted by conduction, or more exactly, by thermal exchange. What state can any vitamins be in after being subjected to an environment in which the water molecules have undergone such manipulation of their atoms? The question is still unanswered as the extremely worrying replies already given have not been sufficiently backed up by science.

Many years of observations will probably be needed before we can say whether this way of cooking is as dangerous as some have said. We had to wait several generations before it was shown that the horizontal barbecue, used since the beginning of time, caused cancer.

If in doubt, therefore, one should be careful and only use the microwave occasionally to reheat food, rather than use it systematically for all home cooking. This is why too frequent use of the microwave by young mothers to heat babies' bottles should be discouraged.

An even better reason to stop this practice is that the baby runs a serious risk of scalding. It is actually difficult to judge the inside temperature of the liquid, which may be boiling hot even when the outside of the bottle is still cold or only luke warm.

It must be added too that the microwave does not sterilise milk, as does normal cooking.

5. Watch out for bad fats

We have seen that some fats, which are called saturated fats, can have a bad effect on the cardio-vascular system. This is the case with butter, cream and meat fats: beef, veal, pork, mutton. Too high a consumption of these foods could therefore lead to a risk of raising the cholesterol level.

The opposite, as we have seen, can be said for other fats which have the property of protecting arteries: fish oil, olive oil, sunflower and also goose and duck fats. In the food choices you make when applying the rules of PHASE I you must always be thinking of how you can balance the various fats.

It would be preferable to limit the amount of meat and meat products to only three times a week, and one of those could be blood sausage, because it is so rich in iron. Substituting poultry (twice a week) and eggs (twice a week) would also be advisable.

6. Some examples of good and bad fat balances

• *Good balance:*

Starter	Sausage	or sardines
Main dish	Fish	or pork chop
Dessert	Cheese	or natural yoghurt

• *Bad balance*

Starter	Ham	or *Frisée aux Lardons* (Green salad with bacon)
Main dish	Steak	or Cutlet with cream (*escalope normande)*
Dessert	Cheese	or *Fromage blanc* with cream

151

Example of two day's meals for Phase I		
Get up 7.10 am	– juice of 2 lemons – 2 kiwis	– juice of 1 grapefruit – 1 pear, 1 kiwi
Breakfast 7.30 am	– cereal (no sugar) – 2 light yoghurts – 1 decaffeinated coffee	– wholemeal bread – unsweetened – jam or marmalade – bowl of skimmed milk
Lunch 12.30	– Greek mushrooms – salmon – small vegetables – cheese	– *crudités* – steak – broccoli – cheese
Tea 4.30 pm	– 1 apple	– 1 apple
Dinner 8.0 pm	– guinea fowl – ratatouille – salad – plain yoghurt	– vegetable soup – wholemeal pasta with – mushrooms – light yoghurt

The rest of the time fish should be selected. Ideally you should have at least three carbohydrate dinners out of seven. You would then have ten meals out of twenty-one (seven breakfasts and three dinners) which did not contain fat and did contain a lot of good carbohydrates.

7. Drinks to be outlawed

Lemonade, fizzy drinks and any reconstituted fruit juices are outlawed as they are generally made from fruit and plant extracts, which are nearly always synthetic and all have one major drawback: they contain a lot of sugar.

They are therefore subject to criticism and have to be totally excluded, especially as the artificial gas also makes them difficult to digest for some people.

Even if they are made from natural extracts, the fizzy drinks should be avoided as they can be toxic.

In natural extracts of citrus fruit it has been seen that there are large traces of bad substances like terpene (an unsaturated hydrocarbon).

As for the worst of them, those based on kola, overflowing with sugar (a bottle of 1.5 litres contains the equivalent of 35 lumps of sugar!), they should either be forbidden, or subject to special labelling (like that found on cigarette packets), reminding users that they can be bad for health.

a. Beer

Beer is a drink that can only be drunk in great moderation. It has no place in either PHASE I or PHASE II.

You don't have to have been to Germany to know what the bad secondary effects of beer are: bloating, bad breath and weight gain.

Unlike wine, beer contains the worst carbohydrates: maltose (glycaemic index of 110) in a concentration of 4 grams per litre.

It must also be noted that association of alcohol with sugar, as in the case of beer, can lead to the appearance of hypoglyceamia which can create tiredness (see Chapter VI, Part I).

b. Spirits

It is obvious that in PHASE I you can draw a line through all distilled alcohol, either as an aperitif (Aniseed, whisky, gin, vodka, etc.) or as pseudo-digestive (Cognac, Armagnac, Calvados, white spirits, etc.).

For an aperitif, you will have to make do with Perrier with a slice of lemon or a tomato juice. In Phase II, we will return to less strict rules when wine, and the most prestigious, Champagne, will be reintroduced.

So, here we are at the end of PHASE I, which, I would repeat, is not *restrictive* in terms of quantity (you must always feel full enough), but which is *selective*. A certain number

153

of foods have been purposely excluded in favour of others, which have better nutritional value.

Do we need to remind you that white bread and anything derived from it (crispbreads, biscuits, toast, etc.) must disappear from the two main meals (when they contain fats), but wholemeal bread and its derivatives must be eaten for breakfast.

If you ate normal amounts of sugar or had quite a sweet tooth before adopting these eating methods, you may lose at least two kilos in the first week. Above all, do not give up at that point, or you will have every chance of regaining what you lost in eight days in only two days.

After this first period, slimming will become more progressive and, to the extent to which you apply our recommendations scrupulously, weight loss will be regular. This loss of weight should then follow a sustained rhythm, even though it is linked to factors which differ in each individual.

PHASE II

This is the phase in which weight will be definitively stabilised. It is all very well to lose weight, but to do so only on a short-term basis proves muddled thinking. Any weight loss which is not thought out in a long term perspective is not only without interest but ill-advised.

Some of the main principles to be respected to stabilise weight are:

1 – You must have a realistic aim, which means that you would be better trying to achieve a reasonable weight that you can maintain rather than aiming at an unrealistic fantasy weight. Going below a BMI of 20 [1] is a mistake. Some women do not seem to have taken this basic assumption to heart!

2 – You have to know how to refuse rationing, which is a source of frustration, because as soon as the "diet" period is over, the body takes its revenge and cannot wait to rebuild its reserve fats. But as you are going to adopt the Montignac Method, which is selective and not restrictive, this trap is not your problem.

-----

1. See Chapter I, Part II.

3 – You have to learn to cope with any psychological upsets. The slimming period is rewarding, but adopting new feeding habits can only be one aspect of fundamentally revising your lifestyle.

4 – You must continue to analyse your relationship to food and understand it. Eating must not be a response to stress (boredom, anxiety, lack of affection). If necessary, complementary steps can be taken with the help of a food behaviour specialist.

You can also continue to do, or decide to learn stress management techniques such as relaxation, sophrology [a] or yoga.

5 – If you have taken up sport to speed up the return of your insulin function to normal, carry on with this physical activity. This will enable you to continue getting your figure into shape, fighting against cellulite and balancing your psyche.

The Montignac Method helps to stabilise weight for several reasons:

- because there are no limits on quantities. At the end of PHASE I there is no risk of a "rebound effect" because the body does not undergo the bad effects of being deprived and then resuming the normal eating cycle;
- the acquisition of good eating habits in PHASE I continues afterwards without stress, especially as wider choices enable you to eat almost everything;
- as PHASE I is easy to accept, the feeling of well-being that it creates prevents the emergence of eating disorders. Because of its educational aspect, it amounts to a veritable behavioural therapy.

If you have applied the precise recommendations given in the last chapter, you should already be genuinely feeling good effects.

---

a. This is a technique often used by sports people, consisting of concentration and relaxation exercises.

However, the risk of resistance, or even opposition by the body to the least change of feeding habits must be noted.

For someone who has really become dependent on bad carbohydrates over the years, it is probable that the body will not accept change readily.

Like alcohol and smoking, here we are often dealing with a real addiction, and in that case, weaning can lead to withdrawal symptoms.

A body that has lived for a long time on constant external glucose input has become a bit lazy, and like a child whose least cry is answered, all it has to do is become hypoglycaemic in order to demand and obtain glucose. Why bother in that case to tire itself making it to keep glycaemia at its normal level?

The act of reducing hyperglycaemia will therefore have as a consequence a limitation of the direct inputs of glucose to that coming from glycogen, thus forcing the body to make glucose from its own reserve fats. Shortly after implementing the principles of the Method which we are proposing, you may find that your body is fighting back by refusing to make its own glucose.

You may then find yourself, fleetingly, in a state of hypoglycaemia with its well-known symptoms, that is, mainly, tiredness.

Don't give in! Don't be tempted to go back to eating something sweet, even temporarily.

It is particularly rather fat people who do sport, who during the first weeks of PHASE I run the risk of coming up against a certain resistance from their body to these new eating habits. There too, the immediate symptom is sudden exhaustion which appears as a feeling of tiredness. If this is only slight, it is best to eat almonds or hazelnuts, which are rich in nutrients.

If the energy loss is more serious you should eat some dried figs or apricots, but in any event some, "good carbohydrates".

The body will quickly understand that you no longer give in easily and that it only has one solution, to reactivate its natural functions, and make its own glucose from its own reserve fats.

Those who have subscribed to low calorie diets and have been dying of hunger for a long time and put on four pounds by just looking at a cake shop window may even have to put up with putting on a little weight, very temporarily, and only about two or three extra kilos.

Actually it is normal that when the body has been subjected to unbearable frustration for years it should be on the alert. It is only natural that when it suddenly receives the minimum amount of energy it normally needed but of which it has always been deprived, it should succumb to the temptation of storing a little, but this will only last for a few days. If this is what happens to you, above all do not give up and go back to starvation rations, as you will only make things worse. On the contrary, persevere.

Your body will very quickly regain confidence and understand that you only wish it well. In a few days you will not only lose that additional weight, but you will begin to see the first results. If you have been following a very strict low calorie diet, you have to slowly increase the calorie ration, at the same time adopting the choices advised in the Method. You will thereby avoid a too rapid change, which is often responsible for temporary weight gain caused by the starving body still thinking in terms of its old low calorie diet reflexes.

It is also possible that you will not lose weight at first, even though you feel slimmer because your body is in better shape. The explanation is that when you stop low calorie diets, your muscular tissue is less dense than it should be (protein deficit). In the first days (or even for a few weeks), a "tissue transfer" occurs, which means a real loss of fat in favour of rebuilding the lean tissues.

158

But we will return to this point in greater detail in **Part II**.

The burning question for any reader now is of course to know how long **PHASE I** will last.

I am tempted to say, at the risk of making you laugh, "for some time!", as it all depends on the amount of weight to be lost, individual sensitivity, and the discipline with which the **PHASE I** principles have been applied.

Return to normal of the pancreatic function, which is the main aim, must be undertaken over a sufficiently long period (a few weeks or months) to enable this to be translated into a lasting improvement of the insulin function.

As an answer must be given to the question, let us say that a minimum of two to three months seems reasonable to us.

But **PHASE II** is in fact only the natural continuation of **PHASE I**, with the possibility of gradually introducing eventual discrepancies [2] which have to be properly managed.

The last chapter in a way served to rid you of your bad eating habits in order to adopt good ones.

You will therefore now be able to operate on the basis of these new reflexes, with a few modifications which allow greater freedom in the application of some of the principles.

Breakfast

Nothing, or almost nothing, will change in relation to our previous recommendations. Continue to follow the principles of always having a big breakfast with wholemeal bread

---

2. The notion of discrepancies was introduced in previous works to signify a deviation from the general principles of the Method – see footnote (4) of this Chapter also.

or wholemeal cereals. If you eat real wholemeal bread, you may spread it with butter or margarine if you like.

You may find when travelling or having a business breakfast, that all you can have is croissants or white bread. Do not worry about having them if it is a special occasion and if you would like to.

If you achieved a good PHASE I, your pancreas should be able to cope with hyperglycaemia without setting off hyperinsulinism and hypoglycaemia as a reaction to it. Sudden fatigue at eleven in the morning should no longer occur.

On the other hand, if you sometimes choose the savoury protein-lipid breakfast, you still should not eat bread, and this is a habit that must never be lost. We will speak of this again when discussing lunch.

Although in PHASE II the occasional discrepancy such as eating a croissant or white bread – may be acceptable, the rule concerning fruit or fruit juice always being eaten before breakfast must be adhered to. An occasional discrepancy must not be confused with a mistake.

Lunch

If lunch is a special occasion (business, family gathering, etc.), you may possibly have an aperitif beforehand. This was not mentioned before as it was excluded in PHASE I.

1. Aperitifs

Several important principles must be respected for aperitifs.

Firstly, the kind of aperitif. It has to have as little alcohol as possible. This is why you should preferably have naturally fermented alcohol and avoid distilled alcohol which is

160

less easily assimilated. Spirits such as whisky, gin, vodka, etc., should therefore be given up.

If you still feel a need, this shows that you are still caught in an alcohol cycle. This explains why people who like spirits drink them without water and on an empty stomach.

As they are more or less hypoglycaemic then, the alcohol will temporarily raise their glycaemia, giving them a passing feeling of well-being.

This habit also tends to lead to the feeling of fatigue which is frequent after a meal.

It is therefore better to drink wine or champagne, or something similar (Saumur made in the Champagne tradition, sparkling wine, etc.).

The fashion of serving a fruity white wine like an *Alsace*, *Sauterne* or even excellent substitutes such as *Monbazillac*, *Barsac*, *Loupiac* or a *Sainte-croix du Mont* as an aperitif should be encouraged.

But for heaven's sake, let's get rid of that regrettable habit of adding a liqueur intended in most cases to mask its mediocre quality, to a white wine, or even worse, to a Champagne. Kir in all its forms should be forbidden, no offence meant to the priest who gave his name to it!

We know that liqueur means sugar, and that sugar plus alcohol lead every time to hypoglycaemia, and therefore to sudden feeling of exhaustion.

The various kinds of punches, ports, sangrias, etc. fall into the same category. These are ideal drinks if you want to feel sleepy and exhausted for the rest of the day or the evening.

Another very important principle to be applied in all cases is not to drink anything on an empty stomach. Except for water. If you stick to the principles of this book, if you become a follower, fight on our side to impose this principle and above all to change habits of the food profession.

Social convention has it that drinks are served first and then, much later, food is brought in, and this latter is often only a possibility. If it should materialise, the food you are given is naturally composed entirely of bad carbohydrates.

If there is only one principle that the reader should learn from this book, it should be that of never drinking any alcoholic beverage on an empty stomach. If this is forgotten, a small metabolic catastrophe is inevitable every time.

Food must therefore be eaten before drinking alcohol, but not just any food.

So that alcohol is not metabolised directly into the blood the stomach must be shut at the level of the pylorus, which is the sphincter situated between the stomach and the beginning of the small intestine. To do this, you have to eat proteins or fats as because they digest slowly this means that the stomach will not be open.

We propose that before drinking any alcoholic beverage you should eat a few cubes of cheese (*gruyère* would be good), or a few slices of *saucisson* or salami type of sausage [3]. This creates a kind of "bowl" made of food, blocking the stomach, which will help, as it were, to neutralise some of the alcohol by partially absorbing it.

By lining the stomach, the fats can also contribute to avoiding, or at least limiting the absorption of alcohol through the stomach wall. It is for this reason too that some claim to counteract the effect of drinking by having a spoonful of olive oil beforehand.

2. Wine

As Doctor Maury says *"Wine has let itself be shut up in a Ghetto, that of alcoholic beverages"* [4].

---

3. Not ordinary sausages as they are full of additives.
4. Doctor Maury, *Le médecine par le vin*, Éditions Artulen, 46 avenue d'Iéna, Paris.

We can only regret that in many instances synthetic sweetened fruit juices have been given precedence over wine, and the consequences for the metabolism are often most regrettable.

If drunk in reasonable quantities (about two or three glasses a day in the middle of the meal), wine is an excellent drink, as it has digestive, tonic, anti-allergic and anti-bacterial qualities. It also contains a large amount of oligo-elements.

As for the aperitifs, wine itself does not cause sleepiness after meals, it is the way in which it is drunk. If you have not already had an aperitif when you sit down in a restaurant, the first thing that the waiter does when you have given your order is to bring the wine, uncork it and fill a glass for each member of the party.

If you drink it, as you are tempted to, you will find yourself in the same state as with the aperitif.

You can do one of two things: either wait to begin eating, or ask for something to eat (cheese, *salami*, olives) to shut the sphincter.

Once seated, you must always wait until you have eaten the starter before beginning to drink any wine.

The longer you wait, the better, as the fuller the stomach the less the bad effects of alcohol will be felt.

Ideally, you should not begin to touch your glass of wine until the middle of the meal.

If you respect this rule you will not only never again feel tired after meals, but in addition you will find it easier to digest.

Drinking wine at meals implies, as we have noted, that the quantity (naturally reasonable) should always be proportional to the amount of food eaten before it.

If you alternate wine and water, the water drunk on top of the wine runs the risk of diluting it and therefore of metabolising it more quickly, whereas it could have been kept prisoner in the food bowl and later absorbed with it during digestion.

It can therefore be concluded that like drinking and driving, a choice must be made between drinking water or drinking wine during a meal, and that it is not advisable to drink water on top of wine.

3. Bread

Even in PHASE II it would be preferable to continue to respect the rule of not having bread during the two main meals.

Bread should be reserved for breakfast. This is the place for your daily bread. Eat as much as you like. Worship it, it deserves it. Go miles to find it. Make it yourself if necessary. Continue to venerate it as a special food, but forget it for the other two meals.

Doing away with bread for the two main meals is still a question of principle. If you managed without it in PHASE I, continue to do so and do not go back on this, except occasionally (discrepancies).

White bread is like cigarettes. When you have got it out of your system you must not start again, otherwise it will take over again.

You have certainly noticed how ex-smokers around you who stopped smoking for a long time have gradually gone back to it. After long abstinence, admired by those around them, they let themselves have a big cigar one day (cigars, they say, have got nothing to do with cigarettes).

And then, as they do not always have big cigars available, they accept little cigars, and then Cigarillos. Then on the day that they do not have any Cigarillos, they go back to cigarettes and are hooked again.

Even wholemeal bread makes a big meal burdened with fats a lot heavier.

164

Do this experiment: have a big meal, with two starters for example, plus a main dish, cheese and even a pudding. If you are following the principles of our Method regarding the composition of the dishes as well as the way of drinking wine, you will feel as light as a feather at the end of the meal, in spite of the large amount of food that you have eaten, and you will digest it without difficulty and will not feel sleepy.

One or two slices of bread on top of such a meal will make you feel disagreeably bloated and upset your digestion.

Do not take the risk of sliding backwards for anything on earth!

If there is one thing that must be forbidden and firmly condemned, it is the deplorable habit that people have when they sit down to table of immediately grabbing the bread (thanks to hypoglycaemia) and even possibly buttering it.

With a glass of wine or an aperitif on an empty stomach, 50 % of your vitality is wiped out for the rest of the day.

Discrepancies

Managing your food intake means managing your weight balance, your fitness and also managing the discrepancies. This means that if you apply the principles of our Method with a certain consistency you can, from time to time, allow yourself a discrepancy, without any bad effect on the general results obtained.

It may be a *soufflé* containing a little white flour, or even fresh pasta, or a small serving of white rice which unexpectedly lands on your plate.

But most often, the discrepancy will be a dessert, as although it is possible to avoid some foods as starters or main dishes, leaving them discreetly aside when you are a guest, it is difficult to categorically refuse dessert, which may contain both sugar and white flour. Once should not be habit forming!

What you have to avoid, however, is multiple discrepancies leading to a situation where you are progressively going back to the old habits.

If you like potatoes and you miss them, once in a while you may spoil yourself. But as with all hyperglycaemic foods, it is important to eat them with fibres so as to limit the rise in glycaemia. If you like chips so much that you are willing to cause a discrepancy, above all do not eat them with meat, eat them with salad. You could even have a whole meal of chips and salad. Then you will have more or less limited the damage.

The same problem arises with carrots. If you wish to eat them, always do so with another food containing a lot of fibre.

In PHASE I the only side dishes that were acceptable were carbohydrates with a very low glycaemic index, with little glucose and a lot of fibres.

In PHASE II you will be able to go back to having low glycaemic index carbohydrates with meat and fish (brown rice, wholemeal pasta, lentils, dried beans, etc.). A *petit salé aux lentilles* (salt pork with lentils) or roast leg of lamb with kidney beans (*gigot aux flageolets*) will be considered as discrepancies. But you can also, as long is it is only occasionally, have a *big* discrepancy which could be something like a side dish with a high glycaemic index (white rice, potatoes).

Some foods were mentioned with reservations in PHASE I, especially for those who had a lot of weight to lose. These were oysters, langoustines and *fois gras*, and these are no longer restricted.

As far as fruit is concerned, naturally we will continue to eat it on an empty stomach in PHASE II. There is one exception that can be made, and that is for red fruit: strawberries, raspberries and blackberries. These fruits can be eaten at the end of a meal, possibly with whipped unsweetened cream.

These in fact run no risk of causing an upset digestion through untimely fermentation.

Dinner

The general principles defined for dinner in **PHASE I** remain the same for **PHASE II**, with the only difference being that some discrepancies can possibly be accepted during dinner instead of and in place of lunch. But be careful, as this does not mean that wide discrepancies can also be permitted for every meal of the day.

The basic rule for good management of discrepancies is precisely accepting or avoiding them by spreading them over time. Too many discrepancies on the same day may risk reliving past experience within the following twenty-four hours, with a return of tiredness, sudden exhaustion and other forms of drowsiness that you had completely forgotten, without mentioning the weight gain of course.

Make a resolution never to accept a discrepancy if it is not going to really give you pleasure in return. Refuse any kind of cheap sweets and chocolates, like those sold in chain stores.

A discrepancy must always be a concession to quality or gastronomy.

Accept a delicious butter croissant made lovingly by an independent baker. Categorically refuse the dreadful industrial products sold in railway stations.

From wholemeal sandwiches to healthy fast food

If you have wholemeal bread to hand, you can always think of making a sandwich with lean meat, smoked salmon or raw vegetables, as long as it is only occasionally.

In the same way, a kind of "fast food" could be invented, where the main dishes (pizzas, tarts, rolls, etc.) would be made from unrefined flours and organic produce.

A "new Hamburger" would in fact be acceptable, retaining its fibres, mineral salts and vitamins and removing sugar, together with most of the saturated fats and pesticide residue.

The organic-dietetic snack of the future might well manage to reconcile the "children of progress" to memories of traditional foods from past generations.

Managing fitness is also managing food. But this new approach to nutrition, as revolutionary, natural and realistic as it is, must not at the same time give rise to compulsive behaviour.

Eating absolutely anything, absolutely anywhere and in absolutely any way, giving in to laziness and commercial exhortation without thought is certainly to be condemned, as it really is irresponsible behaviour.

To become obsessed by nutrition and food quality or paranoid about organic farming should be equally condemned, as it would be going to the other extreme.

The new consciousness that you have acquired about food does not mean that you have to do your shopping exclusively in health food shops, which it must be said do not necessarily guarantee anything. It does not force you to give up the many benefits of modern society, including the consumer society either.

What it should do above all is lead each of you to better discriminate between foods and the choices should from now on be made from a healthier viewpoint.

The quality of the foods we eat, like the quality of the air we breath, conditions our state of health.

Just as we try to get a change of air and a breath of

oxygen, we should look for the greatest diversity in our foods, seek pleasure and enjoyment for our palates, rediscover the varieties of tastes we have lost, cultivate a sacred sense of gastronomy and a respect for what is authentic, natural and pure in the products of our good old mother earth.

Implementation of PHASE II

PHASE II needs more subtle management than PHASE I because it has less strict rules.   In this Phase, there are not, as there were in PHASE I on the one hand the things you cannot do and, on the other, those that you must do.   This is a lot more subtle than that.   You can do everything as long as you do not do too much of it.   Exaggeration is to be outlawed.

The one thing that we must be clear about is that there is no question of going back to old eating habits once results have been achieved as far as slimming and renewed vitality are concerned.   Otherwise, the same causes will lead to the same results, and there is every chance that the weight and tiredness will return.

That means that the basic principles of PHASE I have to be adhered to forever, but maybe applied less rigorously.

During PHASE I, there was no question of discrepancies. PHASE II is precisely the phase of discrepancies.

But you are going to have to manage the discrepancies properly, which means never losing sight of the fact that the principles of PHASE I, apart from small differences, must always be the base you fall back upon.

PHASE II is a phase of freedom, but not just any freedom. It is in fact probationary freedom that must quickly become second nature.

Management of the discrepancies is an art, but it can be

169

done if certain rules are applied. As you know, there are small discrepancies and big discrepancies.

The following are the small discrepancies:

- a glass of wine or champagne as an aperitif after having eaten cheese, *salami* or olives;
- two glasses of wine during the meal;
- a dessert containing fructose (*mousse* or fruit) or a dark chocolate dessert which is rich in cacao [5];
- a dish with good carbohydrates and vegetable oil (a plate of lentils with a few drops of olive oil, a dish of dried beans with a lean meat);
- wholemeal toast with *foie gras* or salmon;
- a slice of wholemeal bread with cheese.

The following are the big discrepancies [6]:

- a glass of aperitif + three glasses of wine with the same meal;
- a starter including a bad carbohydrate (*soufflé*, quiche, flaky pastry);
- a main dish including a bad carbohydrate (sugar, white flour)

In reality, any discrepancy is possible, but it must be understood that all the little discrepancies will be relatively

---

5. See the book *Montignac Recipes and Menus*, which gives a selection of six desserts classified as *"Desserts constituting a slight discrepancy"* and fourteen desserts classified as *"Desserts constituting a very slight discrepancy"*
6. * = slight discrepancy, ** = large discrepancy.

well absorbed by the body if it has completed a good PHASE I and kept to it continuously. Big discrepancies are normally absorbed too, as long as they do not happen too often.

The line on your weighing machine should serve as a warning for you to decide to make changes. It you see that weight is returning, it could be for one of two reasons. Either the pancreas has not yet found an acceptable level of tolerance, or the discrepancies are too frequent. With a little good sense, appropriate measures will be taken as a consequence.

Management of discrepancies is really much easier in real life than you might imagine from the theory.

This is because the consequence of too many discrepancies does not only show as a possible weight gain.

It is generally on the level of your fitness, stamina, or to sum it up, your vitality, that food discrepancies can be best measured. As soon as you have gone a bit too far, you see the consequences on the body so quickly that corrective measures will be taken automatically, one could even say, instinctively.

General rules for PHASE II

1 – Never indulge in two discrepancies in the same meal.

Example:

ACCEPTABLE	UNACCEPTABLE
2 glasses of wine 1 chocolate mousse with more than 70 % cacao	1 aperitif 2 glasses of wine 1 salted pork with lentile *(petit salé aux lentilles)*

2 – *Never have more than one meal with a slight discrepancy in a day.*

This means that in PHASE I for one of the two meals the rules will be stretched

3 – *never have more than one meal in three containing a big discrepancy and one meal in four containing a big discrepancy and two small discrepancies.*

Example:

MEALS WITH A BIG DISCREPANCY	MEALS WITH A BIG DISCREPANCY ** PLUS A SLIGHT DISCREPANCY *
Avocado Hake, broccoli Apple tart ** 1 glass of wine	Oysters Roast lamb, kidney beans * *Profiteroles* ** 3 Glasses of wine

EXAMPLES OF MENUS PHASE II

Breakfast

Fruit
Wholemeal bread + unsweetened marmalade
Light margarine
Decaffeinated coffee
Skimmed milk

Lunch

Avocado *vinaigrette* (oil and vinegar dressing)
Steak with green beans
Crème caramel
Drink: 2 glasses of wine*

Dinner

Vegetable soup
Mushroom omelette
Green salad
Strained *fromage blanc*
Drink: Water

Breakfast

Orange juice
Croissants + *brioches***
Butter
Coffee + milk*

Lunch

Crudités (tomatoes + cucumber)
Grilled Hake fillet
Spinach
Cheese
Drink: one glass of wine only

173

Dinner

Artichokes *vinaigrette*
Scrambled eggs with tomato
Green salad
Drink: Water

DAY N° 3

Breakfast

Fruit
Wholemeal bread
Light butter
Decaffeinated coffee
Skimmed milk

Lunch

Aperitif: + 1 glass of white wine*
Smoked salmon
Led of lamb with kidney beans
Green salad
Cheese
Chocolate mousse*
Drink: 3 glasses of wine**

Dinner

Vegetable soup
Stuffed tomatoes (See *Montignac Recipes and Menus*)
Green salad
0 % fat *fromage blanc*
Drink: water

DAY N° 4

Breakfast

Scrambled eggs
Bacon
Sausage
Coffee or decaffeinated coffee + milk

174

Lunch

A dozen oysters
Grilled tuna with tomato
Strawberry tart**
Drink: 2 glasses of wine*

Dinner

Vegetable soup
Cauliflower with cheese topping (*gratinée*)
Green salad
Yoghurt
Drink: water

DAY N° 5 (Big discrepancy)

Breakfast

Orange juice
Cereal or 0 % fat *fromage blanc*
Coffee or decaffeinated coffee + skimmed milk

Lunch

Foie gras
Grilled salmon + spinach
Fondant with dark chocolate**
Drink: 3 glasses of wine**

Dinner

Cheese *Soufflé*
*Petit salé aux lentilles***
Cheese
*Œufs à la neige**
Drink: 3 glasses of wine**

Note: Day 5 is only given as an example. It is certainly not a recommendation, especially as far as the amount of wine is concerned, which is excessive, as six glasses is over half a litre, which is considered to be the maximum which should not be exceeded in a day. This kind of discrepancy should therefore be very exceptional.

DAY Nº 6 (COMPLETE RETURN TO PHASE I)

Breakfast

Wholemeal bread
0 % fat Fromage blanc
Coffee or decaffeinated coffee

Lunch

Crudités (cucumber, mushrooms, radishes)
Poached Hake with tomato sauce
Cheese
Drink: water, tea or camomile tea

Dinner

Vegetable soup
White ham
Green salad
1 yoghurt

DAY Nº 7

Breakfast

Wholemeal bread
0 % fat fromage blanc + unsweetened marmalade
Coffee or decaffeinated coffee
Skimmed milk

Lunch

Chicory salad
Steak (*entrecôte*) with green beans
Strawberries + unsweetened whipped cream
Drink: 1 glass of wine

Dinner

Fruit
1 orange, 1 apple
1 pear
150 grams of raspberries
Drink: water

Day N° 8

Breakfast

Wholemeal bread
Light butter
Coffee or decaffeinated coffee
Skimmed milk

Lunch

Shrimp cocktail
Tuna + aubergines
Green salad
Cheese
Drink: 2 glasses of wine*

Dinner

Vegetable soup
Plate of lentils
Strawberries
Drink: 1 glass of wine

CHAPTER VI

TIREDNESS: IS FOOD THE CAUSE?

If you sometime you need to see your doctor about feeling tired, it is unlikely that he will question you about your food and even less likely that he will attempt to identify possible vitamin and mineral salt deficiencies.

There is also little chance that he will try to see what food choices could have directly or indirectly led to noticeable general or momentary decline in your fitness.

Hyperglycaemia: too obvious to think of!

A car driver suddenly has to stop at the side of the road. His almost new and well-maintained car has obviously broken down.

When it has been towed to the nearest garage it undergoes a careful mechanical check, but in vain, as nothing can explain the breakdown. When it is moved to a garage specialising in that make of car, the wildest theories are considered. It is taken to pieces, they risk changing some of the main parts and put it back together: it still does not work! And then the problem is finally discovered: it is out of petrol.

Diagnosing hypoglycaemia is a little like running out of petrol: it is too simple to think of.

In the Middle Ages, part of the population had started to cram into the towns with their narrow streets, piled up with garbage and excrement, abounding in pigs, infested with rats and buzzing with flies.

Leprosy, plague, typhoid, cholera, and dysentery then cut down the worthy people for centuries until the day that they hit on the idea that there could be a relationship of cause and effect and that some hygienic measures might be welcome. These terrible plagues have since been called the sicknesses of civilisation, and later smallpox, tuberculosis and even syphilis were to join their number.

If we make a list today of the sicknesses of modern civilisation, we cannot fail to include, amongst others, diabetes, cancer, cardio-vascular diseases, and quite recently, AIDS.

One, however, which is quite characteristic of our times, is easily forgotten: hypoglycaemia.

Even if admittedly it is an affliction that does not kill you, it can however be said to dramatically prevent a full life for those that suffer from it.

1. Glycaemia: hyper and hypo

We saw in the previous chapters that glucose is the fuel of the body, and is particularly needed to make the muscles work, and especially for brain functions.

Without it we die, and if there is not enough this can be seen in various ways, and mainly tiredness.

We know that glucose passes through the blood and that on an empty stomach its average level is around one gram per litre of blood.

To keep the level at this ideal the body successively calls upon two sources of supply:

– glycogen, which constitutes a reserve stock in the liver and muscular tissue;

– production of glucose (neoglucogenesis), which above all comes from the transformation of fats into glucose.

When the sugar (glucose) level increases, as happens after absorption of carbohydrates, a state of hyperglycaemia ensues. When it falls below 0.60 grams per litre, this is called hypoglycaemia.

2. One symptom may lurk behind another

If you have a breakfast made up of good carbohydrates, which means one where the glycaemic index is low, glycaemia will rise within reasonable limits, for example, up to 1.25 g/l, and under the influence of a small insulin secretion, it will gradually return to normal and quickly stabilise again at 1 g/l.

If, on the other hand, breakfast is made up of bad carbohydrates (white bread, honey, jam, sugar, etc.). the glycaemic peak could rise, for example, to 1.80 g/l. Pancreatic secretion of insulin would then be high or even disproportionate, if the pancreas is not in good condition.

In this way, hyperinsulinism would have the effect of abnormally lowering glycaemia, as it could go down as low as 0.45 g/l and thus provoke hypoglycaemia within about three hours of eating.

When glycaemia suddenly goes down, the subject may then complain of symptoms combining paleness, palpitations, sweating, anxiety, trembling, or suddenly feeling extremely hungry. In the worst case, they could faint: this is a classic symptom of hypoglycaemia.

A doctor will easily diagnose this and give the appropriate advice to prevent recurrence, no doubt eliminating any other probability of serious affliction by doing a check-up.

Most individuals who have hypoglycaemia diagnosed, have a tendency to believe that if they are in this state it is probably because they need sugar. But it is exactly the opposite! If, for example, they feel weak at the end of the morning, it is probably following too big an intake of "bad" carbohydrates in a breakfast mainly made up of hyperglycaemic foods.

In other words, if you are hypoglycaemic at 11 o'clock, it is because at 8 o'clock you were hyperglycaemic. This is why this affliction is known as reactive hyperglycaemia. Paradoxically, it is too much sugar that leads to a deficit in glucose, and this is always through an over secretion of insulin. Behind one symptom may lurk another!

3. Functional hypoglycaemia

More often than not, glycaemia goes down gradually and the signs are very ordinary and less easy to diagnose: headaches, yawning, sudden tiredness, lack of concentration, memory lapses, eyesight problems, coldness, but also, according to the person concerned, irritability and aggressivity.

Women also seem to be more prone to this and sometimes suffer more obviously from some symptoms: coldness for example. In offices you may often notice that it is always towards the end of the morning that women feel the need to "put on a cardigan", whereas the temperature has not in fact changed.

Within your family or professional circle it is easy to see that some people get more and more nervous, unstable and even aggressive as mealtime gets closer.

As for yawning and other signs of sleepiness which never fail to enliven participants in business meetings, they too are obvious signs.

A study carried out in France on the subject of accidents occurring on motorways showed that more than 30 % of them were due to a loss of concentration following a fall in glycaemia.

Personnel managers also know well that accidents at work

(in factories or on machines) are always more frequent at certain times of day.

Most of them are linked to lack of concentration, probably related to an abnormal fall in glycaemia.

Symptoms of functional hypoglycaemia are often among the complaints of patients seeing a doctor who think that they are the victims of chronic fatigue or poor circulation of blood to the brain. In reality, these are only the indirect consequences of bad food habits: too much sugar, too much white bread, too many potatoes, too much pasta and white rice, and not enough fibre.

For a long time it was believed that only people with a tendency to put on weight could be subject to hypoglycaemia. Studies have shown that everyone, including thin people, could be effected by this. The difference is found in the metabolism. Some get fat, others do not.

The stupidity of munching bad carbohydrates every time hypoglycaemia occurs, with its symptoms of hunger and sudden tiredness, can readily be judged from this.

Magnates of the agro-food business have not of course been slow to exploit this juicy market by proposing the famous pseudo chocolate bars, which are usually made up of more than 80 % sugar and other glucose ingredients.

Some makes go as far as to speak wrongly of "energy" in their adverts, which may be a little economical with the truth, whilst others promise an immediate energy boost, which is really only the hyper/hypo cycle and is an ideal means of tying the customer into a truly vicious circle.

Eating sweet things, especially between meals, in fact results in maintaining, or even aggravating the situation.

Rise in glycaemia actually happens as quickly and is as marked as fall in glycaemia.

This is precisely the treadmill experienced by victims of snacking. The extreme stage is naturally that in which America is wallowing, constantly eating and drinking hyperglycaemic foods (coke, hamburgers, chips, popcorn, etc.), with the secondary hypoglycaemic consequences that we have already discussed. If they stop the result can be dramatic as they are really caught in a total dependency cycle.

American doctors know of people they call "carbohydrates cravers", which means they are addicted to bad carbohydrates. There is even quite a bit of literature in the States which points to the close link between this "extreme sugar dependency" and violence.

Many studies undertaken particularly in prisons have shown that most delinquents are chronically hypoglycaemic. Other authors go as far as thinking that this is what can explain greater criminality amongst the black population, where poverty leads them to have an even more hyperglycaemic nutrition than the whites. The fact that they are more prone to obesity logically follows.

It has to be realised too that hypoglycaemia is one convincing explanation for alcoholism.

When alcoholic beverages are drunk on an empty stomach they go directly into the bloodstream and immediately cause a rise in glycaemia. This will automatically lead to a large secretion of insulin which will provoke a hyperglycaemic reaction.

It so happens that alcohol, especially for an alcoholic, prevents the release of glucose stored in the liver (glycogen), and makes neoglycogenesis less possible. Thus, one of two things happens, either the alcoholic remains hypoglycaemic, which he cannot stand physically, or he drinks more alcohol to remedy it. It is quite significant that in everyday speech we refer to a "pick-me-up".

The next glass of alcohol will in fact raise glycaemia and the drinker will feel a great sense of relief. From this you will understand the enormous mistake made when trying to disintoxicate an alcoholic of making them drink fruit juices or sweet drinks in place and instead of alcohol, because as long as chronic hypoglycaemia has not been treated, the individual is threatened with a relapse at any time.

Adolescents who kind of "fuel" themselves with coke or

other sweet drinks really find themselves in the same "hyper/hypo" spiral too, and this is probably what explains why they have never been so lymphatic and lazy as they are today.

The more serious result is, as American and French scientists have shown, that adolescents who have been dependent on hyperglycaemic drinks for years are obviously ready to go on to become alcoholic without further transition.

A doctor from a Washington university recently reported that this is what he thinks would explain the dramatic re-emergence of alcoholism on American campuses.

There are many examples of French adolescents who have already accumulated drunken "sprees" by the time they are fifteen, and teachers are well aware of this. It is said that in one small provincial town with a private boarding school the local "black Maria" regularly takes young pupils back to the college on a Wednesday evening in an advanced state of inebriation [1].

In most cases they just smother the affair. It must be said that if you were to try to put the blame where it really belongs, on the "changing food patterns of our society", you would reap nothing but sneers and shrugs.

Nevertheless, "the hunger for the present" felt by our youth, the youth of tomorrow, is satisfied by drinks which create a veritable dependency and "Coke dollars" can be safely laundered by investments in prestige advertising and brilliant marketing strategies.

Sudden tiredness after a meal (post-prandial drowsiness) is a real threat to all those who work. But it should be clear that post-prandial fatigue, as the doctors call it, is the sign of hypoglycaemia! This is a direct consequence of the deplorable way in which meals have been organised, and the worst example of this is certainly "beer and sandwiches".

Contrary to what many people think, it is not necessarily

---

1. Translator's note: French schools have the day off on Wednesday.

185

wine that is the cause of sleepiness, but the way it is drunk, on an empty stomach in most cases. It should also be noted that alcohol increases the effect of sugars, which explains that when it is absorbed with hyperglycaemic foods (white bread, potatoes, pasta, pizza, etc.) it generates hypoglycaemia more quickly. This is why nothing weakens you so quickly as a Kir, beer or whisky-Coke especially when they are drunk on an empty stomach.

What has to be remembered is that most chronic or passing symptoms of fatigue (suddenly feeling worn out) that people suffer from today are linked to hypoglycaemia due to bad nutrition.

We also know that emotional factors can influence glycaemia and manifest themselves in lack of attention leading to abnormal secretion of adrenalin or insulin and thereby to hypoglycaemia.

Before we finish this chapter, it is important to emphasise that hypoglycaemia (and its symptoms) is a relative notion linked to individual sensitivity.

You have certainly noticed that in a room with a constant temperature, some people take clothes off whilst others put on more. This means that at the same temperature some feel cold when others feel too hot.

In the same way, nutritionists have finally accepted the idea that each individual has a personal thermostat and food rations which satisfy the hunger of one person may starve another.

For hypoglycaemia the same applies. This means to say that appearance of symptoms is a biological idea which is entirely relative to one individual or another.

Some people may be near fainting with 0.70 g/l of sugar in the blood, whereas others may feel perfectly fit with 0.50 g/l. This is why it has always been difficult to determine the parameters for the factors which set off hypoglycaemia. Also, the faintness could initially be due to secretion of adrenalin linked to stress for example. If glycaemia is measured at that time it will be normal.

On the other hand, a few hours later, it may be low and therefore responsible for continuing fatigue.

Modern scientific thought is essentially rigorous, and we can only be grateful for this, but it does however have the failing of accepting phenomena as scientifically correct only when it has been possible to verify them statistically, in the same way, using a large number of subjects, as it starts from the premise that everyone is identical. What can be proved with one person must be true for another.

It is because of this basic principle that homeopathy (which is now accepted as an effective therapy for many ailments) has never been officially recognised. It is even rejected, still as a matter of principle, by medical authorities, despite the fact that doctors use it.

Homeopathy cannot in fact be "proved", insofar as it is outside the classical model of scientific control, as it is by its nature founded in individual sensitivity. How can one measure a field with a weighing machine?

Everyone now recognises that variation in blood glycaemia explains most of the symptoms that we have defined, but some still oppose the establishment of a correlation as a matter of principle, as the amounts needed to set it off vary from one individual to another.

Good sense, observation and experience will end by winning out.

Other causes of fatigue

1. Bad macro-nutrient choices

Fatigue can be caused by insufficient input of proteins.
A diet which is too restrictive or badly balanced may

187

actually be deficient in proteins. This relative deficiency may have several consequences:

- weight gain because of metabolic troubles;
- muscular wasting, from which stems a feeling of fatigue at the least effort;
- slowing of growth in children.

Excessive fats in a meal can also lead to a fall in energy.
Excess fats considerably slow digestion which can last for four or five hours. This leads to a disagreeable heavy feeling in the stomach and to drowsiness.

2. Micro-nutrient deficiencies

Vitamin B deficiency can also lead to the appearance of fatigue. This is readily observable in alcoholics, pregnant women who vomit and sports people.
You should know that the B vitamins, which are water soluble, easily disappear in the cooking water of vegetables and starches, and this should therefore be kept to make soup.

Other causes of fatigue due to a deficiency in micro nutrients:

- when the level of vitamin B6 in the blood is lowered by taking the pill;
- when vitamin B9 (or folic acid) is not present in sufficient quantity, as is the case of pregnant women and the elderly;
- when vitamin B12 is deficient, as is often the case with vegetarians;
- Vitamin C deficiency is often a worry for smokers and people who do not eat enough fruit and raw vegetables. This deficiency also predisposes towards infection and prevents absorption of iron;
- magnesium, if lacking, can lead to "spasmophilia" and greater vulnerability to stress;

– iron deficiency, which is very frequent in women, is the source of anaemia, infection and fatigue;
– antioxidant deficiency (beta-carotene, C and E vitamins, zinc and selenium) makes it difficult of fight free radicals which are responsible for premature ageing, cardio-vascular diseases and cancer.

3. Bad management of alcoholic beverages

The way an alcoholic beverage is drunk may have repercussions on energy levels. This is why you should never drink alcohol on an empty stomach, as it could lead to migraines, giddiness or various accidents (at work, driving) through lack of concentration. Excess alcohol during meals has the same results.

Women seem more sensitive than men to the same quantities of alcohol, because their enzyme system is less efficient at the level of the liver.

As a secondary effect, alcohol leads to dehydration because it increases perspiration and has a diuretic effect.

As it happens, 1 % dehydration lessens muscular strength by 10 %. At 2 %, muscular strength goes down 20 %. From this stems a feeling of fatigue which is abnormal, if it is not caused by intense physical exercise.

4. Over-sensitivity to nutritional pollution

The effects of absorption of massive doses of pesticides, herbicides, fungicides, nitrates, antibiotic residues, lead and mercury on the body over several decades are not well known.

However, cases of poisoning by beta-agonists from offal, allergy to some dyes, without mentioning diarrhoea from salmonella and a few rare epidemics of listeria and trichi-

Table of vitamins

Vitamin	Role	Sources	Added risk factors	Defficiency symptoms
A Retinol	Growth Eyesight Skin condition	Liver, egg yolk, milk, butter, carrots, spinach tomatoes apricots	Smoking Drinking Contraceptive pill Viral hepatitis Barbiturates	Poor night vision Sensitivity to light Dry skin Skin sensitivity to sunlight Susceptibility to ear, nose and throat infections
Provitamin A Beta-carotene	Protection against cardi-vascular disease, ageing and cancer	Carrots, cress, spinach, mango, melon, apricots, broccoli, peaches, butter		
D Calciferol	Mineralisation of bones and teeth : metabolism of calcium phosphate	Liver, tunas, sardines, egg yolk, mushrooms, butter, cheese, Sunshine	Lack of sunlight Over-use of total sunscreen creams Elderly people who do not go out	Children : rickets Elderly : osteomialisis (osteoporosis = demineralisation of bones
E Tocophenol	Anti-oxidant against free radicals and protection of polyunsaturated fatty acids Protection against cardio-vascular disease and prevention of some cancers	Oils, hazelnuts, almonds, whole cereals, milk, butter, eggs, dark chocolate, wholemeal bread		Muscular fatigue, risk of cardio-vascular disease Ageing skin
K Menadione	Blood coagulation	Made by intestinal bacteria Liver, cabbage, spinach, eggs, broccoli, meat, cauliflower	Long-term antibiotic treatments Over-use of laxatives Premature baby	Haemorrhages (bleeding)
B1 Thiamine	Neuro-muscular functions Metabolism of carbohydrates	Yeast wheat germ, pork, offal, fish, whole cereals, wholemeal bread	Food intake tending to hyperglycaemia Diabetes Drinking Pregnancy Diuretics	Fatigue, irritability, Memory loss Lack of appetite Depression, muscle weakness
B2 Riboflavin	Metabolism of carbohydrates, fats and proteins Cell ventilation Vision	Yeast, liver, kidneys, cheese, almonds, eggs, fish, milk, cocoa	Drinking Not eating enough milk products and cheese	Seborrhoea Acne rosacea Photo phobia Brittle, lifeless hair Lip and tongue sores
PP or vitamin B3, or niacin, or nicotinic acid	Provides energy through oxide-reduction	Dried yeast, bran, liver, meat, kidneys, fish, wholemeal bread, dates, pulses Intestinal flora	Drinking Anti-Parkinson disease treatment Vegetarian diet, too much maize	Fatigue, insomnia, anorexia, skin and mucous membrane lesions

190

VITAMIN	ROLE	SOURCES	ADDED RISK FACTORS	DEFFICIENCY SYMPTOMS
B5 Pantothenic acid	Aids many energy metabolism functions Skin, hair and mucous condition	Dried yeast, kidneys, eggs, meat, mushrooms, cereals, pulses	Drinking High intake of preserved and frozen foods	Fatigue Nausea, Headaches Vomiting, Psychoses Low blood pressure Posture problems Hair loss,
B6 Pyridoxine	Protein metabolism Lecithin synthesis Present in 60 enzyme systems	Yeast, wheat germ, Soya, liver, kidneys, meat, fish, brown rice, avocados, pulses, wholemeal bread	Taking the Pill Drinking	Fatigue, Depression Irritability Dizziness Nausea Skin lesions Craving for sweet things Headaches due to glutamates
B8 Biotin	Present in many cellular reactions	Intestinal flora Yeast, liver, kidneys, chocolate, eggs, mushrooms chicken, cauliflower, pulses, meat, wholemeal bread	Long-term taking of antibiotics, Too many raw eggs	Fatigue, loss of appetite Nausea, muscle fatigue Greasy skin, Hair loss Insomnia, depression Neurological problems
B9 Folic Acid	Protein metabolism Cell manufacture	Yeast, liver, oysters, Soya, spinach, cress, green vegetables, pulses, wholemeal bread	Drinking, pregnancy Old age Many medicines Cooking methods Anaemia	Fatigue, Memory loss, Insomnia, depression, Mental confusion in elderly Slow healing Neurological problems
B12 Cyanocobalamine	Red corpuscle synthesis Enzyme reactions Skin and nerve cell condition	Liver, kidneys, oysters, herrings, fish, meat, eggs	Vegetarian diet Cobalt deficiency	Fatigue, irritability, Paleness, anaemia, loss of appetite, sleep disorders, Neuromuscular aches Loss of memory, depression
C Ascorbic Acid	Many tissue and cell metabolism roles, (iron absorption) Traps free radicals, Formation of collagen and conjunctive tissue Anticorp formation Synthesis of L-Carnitine Combats stress	Rosehips, black currant, parsley, kiwis, broccoli, green vegetables, citrus fruits, liver, kidneys	Smoking Lack of fruit and raw vegetables in the diet Macrobiotic diet Stress Long-term infection	Fatigue, drowsiness Loss of appetite Muscular aches Lower resistance to infection Breathlessness on exertion

191

nosis which have already been seen. In every one of these cases the symptoms also include some fatigue.

This is why it is important to choose, if possible, foods from organic farms as they have more micro-nutrients and do not contain undesirable chemical products.

CHAPTER VII

PREVENTION OF CARDIO-VASCULAR DISEASE

Modern urban populations (men as well as women) statistically run a high risk of cardio-vascular disease.

Every year about 110 000 people suffer from coronary thrombosis and 50 000 deaths can be attributed to coronary arteriosclerosis.

However, even though this figure is high in relation to the population, France is at the tail end just before Japan, which has the lowest score. This is in fact three times less than the United States, four times less than Finland (the country most at risk), and far behind the United Kingdom, Canada, Norway and Germany.

Though hypercholesterolemia is a risk factor that many studies have been able to highlight, there are others which are even more important: smoking, high blood pressure, heredity, diabetes, *and all the things we are probably not yet aware of"* say the specialists.

Everyone is aware that cardio-vascular diseases are the most frequent cause of death in the world. But, as Professor Apfelbaum loves to remark, we often do not realise that the average age of death by cardio-vascular disease is between seventy and seventy-five years of age, which means that it is close to the average life expectancy today.

> ## Cardio-vascular risk is different for men and women
>
> *For men, it is around 35 to 55 years old. Women, on the other hand, are protected by their hormones until the menopause.*
>
> *After that, only those not on hormone replacement therapy are exposed.*
>
> *The risk only becomes clear at about seventy years old with arterial ageing.*

In addition, all the international studies show that wherever lower cholesterol (a risk factor) has been achieved mortality from coronary thrombosis has been reduced, but most surprisingly total mortality has not gone down proportionately.

This is exactly what has happened in the States, where a huge anti-cholesterol campaign has been waged since 1985 which now shows up in behaviour close to hysteria or paranoia such as only the Americans could provoke.

There they have tried everything to reduce the particularly high level of cardio-vascular disease. *"Every eighty seconds, an American will die of a heart attack"* Dr. Lenfant emphasised. It should be pointed out that forty million adult Americans have a cholesterol level far above normal.

A committee of experts has been created, with the aim of formulating "recommendations", by some ten or so professional medical associations, insurance companies, pharmaceutical industries and agro-food businesses.

Their advice has been widely publicised, with great media support, to the various sectors of the population. Brochures intended to educate patients were distributed through fifty thousand doctors. Special classes were given to dieticians and nurses, as well as to other health professionals.

This vast campaign, entitled *"know your cholesterol numbers"* has of course influenced American living habits. It must be said that at the same time the food industry has rushed to exploit this new "no cholesterol" market. This means that anything with the least amount of fat in it has had the intruder removed. Butter, now called *"I can't believe it isn't butter"* is just like its famous cousin *Canada Dry*; "it looks like butter, it tastes like butter, but it isn't butter". It is just one more synthetic product, replacing it with a pseudo-substitute.

Pork products and cheese amongst other things are the object of the same industrial interference. Fats are removed and it is all stuck back together attractively, with the advantage for the consumer that they have the taste of the fats without having them.

Professor Slama, who condemns such manipulation, is right to believe that the human body will not let itself be misled without reacting in one way or another. When you know the complexity of the many mechanisms which start up as soon as food is eaten, right from the first taste (neurotransmitters, hormones, enzymes) we can fear the worst kind of imbalances.

These practices are even more suspect to the French eye as their traditional and authentic food, which has an added gastronomical bonus, is amongst the best in the world as far as coronary mortality statistics are concerned.

But, this is not reason enough to neglect hypercholesterolemia. Without turning it into an obsessive refrain, as it is in the States, we should nevertheless objectively assess implications for our health and see what simple precautions in regard to food may be adopted to guard against it.

Cholesterol is good for your health!

Cholesterol is not necessarily the intruder we may believe. On the contrary, it is an indispensable substance for our bodies.

It must be pointed out too that it derives from two sources: 75 % is synthesised by the liver, which means it is made by the body itself, and only 30 % comes from food.

Another way of putting it is that you may very well have a diet without any external input of cholesterol (if you only eat boiled carrots for example), and still find that you have a high and critical blood cholesterol level for other reasons. This is what makes professor Apfelbaum say that *"food cholesterol and blood cholesterol only have a very weak link, and in some people none at all"*.

Cholesterol is in fact an indispensable molecule for the building of cell membranes, certain hormones, and making bile. It transits in the blood by proteins which act as a kind of "transporter". There are two categories:

– *low density lipo-proteins*, LDL's, which distribute cholesterol to the cells and especially those of the arterial walls which fall prey to these fat deposits.

This is why LDL-cholesteral has been christened "bad cholesterol" because it coats the inside of the blood vessels in the long run and they become blocked.

This blocking of the arteries can lead to cardio-vascular illnesses because of:

• Inflammation of the arteries in the lower limbs;
• angina or coronary thrombosis;
• cerebral vascular problems, possibly leading to paralysis;

– *high density lipo-proteins* or HDL's, which take the cholesterol to the liver which eliminates them.

HDL-cholesterol is called "good cholesterol" as it does not build up in the veins. On the contrary, it has the

196

property of cleaning the arteries of arteriosclerosis deposits. You will easily understand then that the higher the HDL, the lower the risk of cardio-vascular illness.

Levels in the blood

Present standards are much stricter than those used for many years. Three points have to be noted:
1 – total cholesterol must be below or equal to 2 grams per litre of blood;
2 – LDL cholesterol must be lower than 1.3 g/l;
3 – HDL cholesterol must be above 0.45 g/l in men and 0.55 g/l in women.

Cardio-vascular risk

Cardio-vascular risk is twice as high if the cholesterol level is 2.2 g/l and four times as high if it is over 2.6 g/l. But, it has been observed that 15 % of coronary thrombosis occurs in subjects with a total cholesterol level below 2 g/l. This is why this theory is of only relative significance.

What is most important is the amounts of LDL and HDL, and above all the ratio of total cholesterol to HDL, the cholesterol must be lower than 4.5. Forty-five percent of the French have levels above normal and about eight million have a total cholesterol level over 2.5 g/l. The importance of taking this question seriously can be seen if you realise that lowering cholesterol by 12.5 % makes it possible to reduce the level of coronary thrombosis by 19 %.

Necessary dietary changes

In cases of hypercholesterolemia, the doctor can prescribe certain treatments, but this must be as a last resort.

In most cases good food management should prove sufficient.

Here then is the advice that you may follow to lower your cholesterol level, if it is too high, but also as a safeguard for the future.

1. Lose weight

It has been observed that slimming (where there is excess weight), in most cases leads to an improvement of all the biological parameters. Lowering the cholesterol level is certainly the first visible improvement, on condition, of course, that you do not make the mistake of eating excessive amounts of bad fats.

2. Limit input of cholesterol from food

Some foods have a high level of cholesterol, such as egg yolk and offal. For a long time, the WHO (World Health Organisation) advised not going above a daily input of 300 mg per day. However, recent work has proved that, paradoxically, this aspect of diet is very secondary and that a food input of 1 000 mg of cholesterol a day would only lead to an increase of about 5 % of cholesterolemia.

Recent publications have shown that eggs have much less effect than it was long thought. It would seem in fact that the large amount of lecithin in them neutralises their cholesterol content.

You can then forget the amount of cholesterol in foods, but on the other hand you must take account of the degree of saturation of the fatty acids consumed.

3. Choose your lipids (fats)

As we saw in the chapter on the nutritional composition of foods, fats should be classified into three categories.

a. Saturated fats

These are those found in meat, pork products, eggs, milk, milk products, cheese and palm oil, and also nowadays in biscuits, cakes and pastries.

These fats theoretically raise the total and above all the LDL-cholesterol level, and this is deposited on the arterial walls and can lead to vascular problems.

As for poultry, as long as the skin is removed, the saturated fat level is low. Eating it should, therefore, have little effect on the level of cholesterolemia.

b. Poly-unsaturated fats of animal or vegetable origin

– Poly-unsaturated fatty acids of animal origin are mostly contained in the fat of fish.

For a long time it was thought that Eskimos, whose diet is largely composed fish fats, did not get cardio-vascular diseases for genetic reasons. Then it was realised that it was precisely the nature of their food that was the best prevention factor.

Eating fish fats actually leads to a lowering of LDL-cholesterol and triglycerides, and it also makes the blood more fluid which means there is less of a risk of thrombosis.

From this you will understand that contrary to what was believed for a long time, the more fatty the fish, the more beneficial its effect on cholesterol. The consumption of salmon, tuna, mackerel, anchovies and herrings must therefore be encouraged.

– Poly-unsaturated fatty acids, of vegetable origin, were given pride of place for a long time, as they lower total cholesterol. But it was noticed that though they did in fact lower LDL-cholesterol (a desirable effect) they also lowered HDL cholesterol, which is not a good thing.

They are found in sunflower, rapeseed, walnut and grapeseed oils. They are in addition very prone to oxidation, and we know that an oxidised oil is dangerous for the arteries.

The same should be said when they are turned into mar-

199

garine as a recent study of 17 000 American nurses showed that margarine actually helps fat to deposit in the blood vessels.

c. Mono-unsaturated fats

These are the ones that should be preferred. The best amongst them is oleic acid, found notably in olive and rapeseed oils.

It may be affirmed that olive oil is world champion of all the fats which have a beneficial effect of cholesterol. It is effectively the only one that manages to lower bad cholesterol (LDL) and increase the good (HDL).

From this, some of you will have understood that tuna with olive oil thereby becomes a veritable antidote to cholesterol.

We also now know that goose and duck fat, especially when they have been fattened to produce *foie gras*, belong in this category of mono-unsaturated fatty acids.

Foie gras, *magrets* and other goose and duck preserves can therefore be eaten with a good conscience, as they have a beneficial effect on the cardio-vascular system.

4. Increase your intake of food fibres

The presence of fibres in the digestive tubes actually improves the metabolism of fats.

It has also been noted that consumption of pectin (through eating apples for example) leads to a noticeable lowering of cholesterol level, and this is also the case for all soluble fibres, such as gums from white beans, or those contained in seaweed (alginates).

5. Drink a little wine

Professor Masquelier has shown that alcohol increases the level of "good cholesterol" (HDL-cholesterol) and that the polyphenols it contains protect the arterial walls.

It is evident from the statistics that the countries where the population regularly drinks wine (France, Italy, Spain, Greece, etc.) are amongst those with the lowest level of mortality from cardio-vascular diseases.

6. Improve your lifestyle

Stress, smoking and a sedentary life also have negative impact on cholesterol and the arteries. Better living is imperative, therefore, not only as a way to cure problems but also as a preventive measure.

The Mediterranean diet

This constitutes the best cardio-vascular protection possible, as it associates:
– lots of fish (but little meat)
– vegetables and especially onions;
– pulses (white beans, lentils, broad beans, chick peas)
– fruit: citrus fruits and nuts (walnuts)
– high fibre bread;
– fermented milk products (yoghurt);
– garlic;
– olive oil (but little butter);
– wine.
   Crete, where the people drink wine and use a lot of olive oil, is the European region where the level of cardio-vascular disease is the lowest.

---

7. Think of reducing hyperinsulinism

Many American doctors are astonished at the fact that doing away with cholesterol in food, as well as doing away with fats, does not necessarily lead to a substantial reduction of cholesterol levels in their patients.

It has however been shown that when a diet with a low glycaemic index was adopted it did lead to less hyperinsulinism, which itself invariably optimised the regulation of blood parameters (cholesterol, triglycerides), although, paradoxically, fat and cholesterol intake from food were not diminished. In some cases they even increased.

Doctor Morrison C. Bethea, Surgeon and Cardiac specialist at the big Mercy Baptist Hospital in New Orleans was able to verify this statistically with his patients after he had adopted the Montignac Method in his Department.

8. Prevent excess triglycerides in the blood

Even taken in isolation, this anomaly is now recognised as a cardio-vascular risk factor in its own right. It is most often due to excess alcohol or sugar. On a practical level therefore you must:

– eat fatty fish more often;
– have carbohydrates with a low glycaemic index;
– avoid sweet things and alcoholic beverages.

9. All you need to know

According to Professor Serge Renaud, a specialists in fats, and Director of Research at INSERM (the French National Institute for Scientific Research), some studies would seem to show that, in cheese, fatty saturated acids which are responsible for cholesterol form insoluble salts in combination with calcium which are badly absorbed by the intestine. Eating cheese would therefore be much less risky for cholesterol than it had been thought until now.

Other studies also show that fermentation of cheeses made from unpasteurised milk, which happens naturally, leads to a veritable transformation of the nature of the fats. The

202

molecular structure of the saturated fat is in fact modified to the extent of completely neutralising absorption by the intestines.

Traditional cheeses, from unpasteurised milk, probably do not have any adverse effects on the cardio-vascular system (see diagram below).

Food fats (lipids) are made up of 98 % triglycerides formed by the combination of one alcohol molecule (glycerol) and three fatty acid molecules.

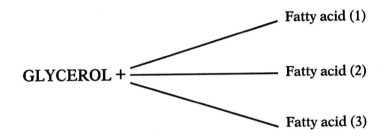

Amongst the saturated fats, only the fatty acids in position 2 are well absorbed by the wall of the intestine. As it happens, natural fermentation of unpasteurised milk, which modifies the molecular structure of the fats largely removes the fatty acids in position 2.

Thus, even if the amount of saturated fats is high in an unpasteurised cheese, the amount absorbed by the intestine is reduced. It should also be mentioned that a high level of cholesterol, even when the amount of saturated fat consumed is low, can be linked to a deficiency in vitamin PP.

Summary of the measures to be implemented for those with hypercholesterolemia

- *Lose weight, if you are fat.*
- *Lower your meat intake (Max.: 150 grams a day).*
- *Chose lean meats (poultry, lean beef).*
- *Replace them more often with poultry (without the skin).*
- *Avoid fatty pork products and offal.*
- *Choose fish (at least 300 grams a week)*
- *Do not eat much butter (Max. 10 grams a day) and margarine.*
- *Have skimmed milk and 0 % fat milk products. Eat Yoghurts.*
- *Increase intake of fibres (fruit, cereals, vegetables and pulses).*
- *Increase consumption of mono and poly-unsaturated vegetables (olive, sunflower, rapeseed, maize).*
- *Make sure you eat enough vitamins A, PP, C and E, selenium and chrome (beer yeast).*
- *Drink (possibly) wine rich in tannin (max. 1/2 bottle per day), as it contains polyphenols.*
- *Keep a watch on your stress level.*
- *Possibly take up an endurance sport.*
- *Stop smoking.*

CHAPTER VIII

NUTRITION AND SPORT

If by chance you should be walking the streets of New York well before the first light of day, from five in the morning onwards, you will not fail to notice the American joggers, sweating blood and water dressed in their appropriate little outfits.

In spite of the extreme pollution level which their stimulated lungs are happily taking advantage of, these early bird sportsmen and women are sacrifices to a ritual which is henceforth written into the manual of the perfect American citizen.

Apart from a few histrionic marathon runners, most of the battalions of these early morning "non-losers" are actually made up of people who think that only a big daily physical effort will maintain the dream of fitness and above all prevent them from becoming obese couch potatoes like much of the rest of their nation.

America has for years now fallen into step and, in spite of the rise in average weight, Americans are still convinced that the best way of slimming is to watch calories on the one hand and use lots of energy on the other.

Parisians, who are much more reasonable, are quite happy for their part, to do a few turns round the lake in the Bois de Boulogne on a Saturday morning, and this is more with a view to getting a weekly breath of fresh air as well as an excuse to meet up with their friends. In addition, many of them continue to stretch their muscles afterwards with a substantial very French meal, if only to regain the energy that they have not necessarily lost!

In 1989, a poll done by a big French weekly indicated that 66 % of the French think that the best way of slimming is to do a sport.

This is in fact a preconceived idea that is even more surprising as most of those who have tried it have not been successful, because the idea of losing weight by exercise without a change of eating habits is a total illusion.

It cannot however be denied that sport increases energy expenditure, but the expenditure is really much lower than one would imagine.

The work of Dr. Mondenard has effectively shown that many hours have to be spent on it in order to lose one kilo.

This demonstrates that someone who wants to lose five kilos in four months just doing sport would have to do one and a half hours of jogging five times a week.

SPORT UNDERTAKEN REGULARLY	TIME NEEDED TO LOSE 1 KILO OF FAT BY DOING A SPORT	
	MEN (Hours)	WOMEN (hours)
Normal walking	138	242
Fast walking	63	96
Golf	36	47
Bicycle	30	38
Leisure swimming	17	21
Jogging	14	18
Tennis	13	16
Squash	8	11

It's stamina that counts!

What all candidates for physical exercise have to realise is that if the exercise is continued beyond a certain limit weight loss results do ensue. So, one continuous hour of muscular exercise will be more effective than three times thirty minutes on the same day.

When resting, the body uses the fatty acids circulating in the blood as a fuel as well as the ATP from the muscles.

As soon as intense physical exercise begins, it will "pump" out glycogen from the muscles, and the latter would be used up within about twenty minutes if this was all you could rely on.

After the first twenty-five minutes exercise, half the energy used will come from glycogen, and the other half from the transformation of reserve fats (lipolysis).

Then, after forty minutes exercise, it is mostly the fats which are used, in order to conserve the remaining glycogen. It is therefore after forty minutes of sustained continuous exercise, of almost maximum intensity, that the reserve fats start to melt.

If we say, hypothetically, that you do three times twenty minutes of leisure sports in a day, it will then be clear that the fuel source for this is glycogen, and it has time to be renewed from subsequent food after each session.

To get convincing results, an endurance sport (bicycle, jogging, swimming, etc.) should be practised at least three times a week, keeping up the exercise for a minimum duration of forty minutes. Interrupting this for three days will cancel out all the results previously obtained.

In addition, the sportsman or woman should adopt eating habits in conformity with the principles laid down in this book, and especially to prevent any risk of hypoglycaemia [1].

---

1. High level sport requires a much more complex nutrition and relies on other nutritional rules which vary for each sport, and these are too detailed to be mentioned in this book.

It is also necessary to start slowly, avoiding a sudden increase in the time spent on the exercise without any previous training. The body needs to get used to it in gradual stages so that its physiological functions adjust.

Sport can be good for you!

It can in fact be beneficial if undertaken intelligently, with the main aim being to achieve a healthier lifestyle and oxygenate the body.

It may almost be said in fact that the human body (like each of its functions) "only really wears out if it is not used".

Physical exercise is therefore a kind of constant renewal which helps, amongst other things, to fight against ageing by improving the heart and lung functions.

Even if weight remains the same when you exercise, fat is gradually replaced by muscle, and your figure will become neater.

Muscular activity may also be an effective help in "overhauling" the body, that is to say in the "renovation" that the recommendations in this book are calculated to bring about.

Another thing that must be noted is that glucose tolerance is improved and hyperinsulinism (a factor contributing to hypoglycaemia and obesity) is reduced perceptibly. It is above all through this that sport is useful as it speeds up the correction of hyperinsulinism.

It may be added that high blood pressure, and also hypercholesterolemia, are clearly improved, if these conditions were present [2].

On the psychological level, a reasonable amount of sport can be very rewarding, even if only because you discover your own body and get a real impression of feeling somewhat

---

2. A man over forty *must* have a cardio-vascular examination with an electro-cardiogram showing him exercising before undertaking a sport.

younger. Maybe at first you will feel it as an imposition, but it will quickly become a real source of well-being as your fitness improves.

After you have lost weight, the general improvement in the metabolism brought about by physical exercise could be an additional guarantee of weight stabilisation and sustained fitness.

Don't go off on the wrong track

In our society, attitudes are unhappily a little too extremist as regards sport. Between the smoking pseudo-sportsman, "alcoholic" who spends most of his time, and the breaks in the football in the pub or in front of the tele, and the middle-aged lady-killer who is killing himself to keep young by trying to emulate professional sportsmen, there is a just milieu, which only experience will teach you.

Absenteeism on a Monday morning is not only due to hangovers and other eating excesses over the weekend, but can also be put down to the imprudence of many who, without any previous experience and training, and without enough liquids, have, starry-eyed, misjudged their real capabilities.

Healthy management of food, as well as keeping up reasonable and regular physical activity, these are the necessary conditions to be able to face the mounting years tranquilly, youthfully and optimistically. But this is also a state of mind.

When you see some people obstinately waiting five minutes for a lift to go up to the first floor, or jumping in their car to go and get cigarettes at the corner shop, you can only feel the same pity as you would for someone who only lives on hamburgers and coke.

PART II

Woman is a delicate creature! Anyway, that idea that has always prevailed, to the point that they have been called "the weaker sex".

However, scientists now assure us that she has greater stamina than man, and not only because her life-expectancy is greater.

Man, we are told, would be physically incapable of supporting the trial of childbirth and women would paradoxically seem to have greater stamina than men even if they are delicate.

In reality, women are above all more sensitive, but also more complex. Their lives are governed by a complicated hormonal system which, from puberty to menopause, and through maternity, submits their body to many transformations.

Like an extremely sophisticated engine, the female body is sensitive to the least change. This is why it has a more finely tuned regulatory system and, as a consequence, is more vulnerable to bad treatment.

Once you know this, you can understand better why women are "really" more sensitive to the medicines administered to them by men and why the possible side effects are more marked.

Finally, you can understand even better why this extreme

sensitivity, when coupled with bad eating habits, has consequences which are even more evident on the weight level, because they are aggravated by hormonal upheavals.

After having indicated in Part I the nutritional rules that should generally be adopted for permanent weight loss and better health, I propose in Part II that we should now look at how women can apply them to get the best results.

CHAPTER I

VARIATIONS ON AN IMAGE:
THE FEMALE BODY

Let's imagine that we are living in the year 2500 and contemporary historians have decided to research the shape of the female body in the XXth century. When they have gone through the many women's magazines of the time and noted the many photos in them, all featuring lanky figures, with one thing in common, their slimness or even thinness, these observers from the future would surely come to the conclusion that everyone was like this at the time.

We make exactly the same mistake today when we study the *Three Graces* by Raphaël, Rubens' *Sirens*, or nearer to our time, Renoir's nudes, Maillol's sculptures or Courbet's *"Bathers"*. The least that can be said is that all these works of art show women who are well built and it would be logical to think that historically all women were as plump and well covered.

It would be more pertinent to wonder if the painters in the past were trying to reflect the reality of the time in their work, or if they were rather hoping to show a certain "feminine" ideal.

In the same way, modern women's magazines are now obviously trying to develop the image of an atypical female body which is in fact only the projection of their readers' dreams.

Canons of beauty

We actually worship the rare and exceptional. In days gone by fatness was a sign of social success: it signified that your table was "well spread" every day and that you had sufficient means to be able to eat copiously. Being slim or thin (the word "emaciated" was used at the time) was only too common.

This is why more generous figures and opulent plumpness corresponded to the prevailing canons of beauty, as they were the exception.

It should also be noted that food supplies in the past were random for the majority of the population. Wars, peasant revolts and bad harvests could at any moment lead to scarcity or even famine. To be able to eat enough not to go hungry every day was a luxury, and this is why if you were lucky enough to be covered in fat this in fact constituted a precious reserve should circumstances mean that food was rationed.

When people were overweight, this was a bit like a "comprehensive insurance policy" against hazardous harvests and it did not have the negative implications it has today. It was considered an even more valuable guarantee as it was uncommon.

A little extra weight was, in the past, also thought to be a criterion of good health and as a consequence of strength. In other words, a well-covered woman could only be a good child-bearer whose generous haunches would have no difficulty in accommodating a promising pregnancy. This idealised picture of woman is still prevalent in a certain number of third world countries.

To explain the evolution of the female æsthetic, sociologists have a tendency to say that beauty canons have progressively evolved with changing fashions.

Others are more of the opinion that fashion has never

done more than be in the forefront of a movement that was only waiting for a "means" of expressing itself.

Paul Poiret's influence at the beginning of the century would therefore certainly have contributed to tipping the balance when he proposed doing away with corsets.

After that, women no longer tried to hide their bodies under voluminous clothes or rely on a multitude of artifices. On the contrary, their dresses would mould their figures and underline their curves. A few years later, with the help of the women's liberation movement, they went as far as to deny the principles of femininity by proposing quasi-androgynous models.

The disquiet of the masculine gender faced by feminine sexuality, suddenly highlighted by Freudian analysis, was to have even greater repercussions on our ideas. Eroticism gradually tended to disappear from paintings and some painters did not hesitate to "assassinate" the female body, depicting it as emaciated or with geometrical shapes, as did Picasso and Buffet.

At the same time as these socio-cultural phenomena were taking place, two other factors were going to be crucial in giving even more weight to slimness: plumpness and even obesity became generalised in a trend-setting country like America, and in addition doctors discovered that overweight was actually a serious risk factor for health.

Women who think fat

To have a "normal" body, insofar as such normality can be defined (as it is often an individual impression), is a legitimate desire for any woman. The difficulty is that a lot of women set their sights too high, or rather a little low, thinking that the models in their favourite magazines are tallies where the 36, 24, 36 measurements are written in stone.

Our culture is one of standardisation and as soon as you do not match the recognised criteria you are quickly labelled as belonging to the hordes of eccentrics, "uglies", and consequently unlovable people.

A young girl who does not match up to the "norm" undoubtedly thinks that no boy will find her desirable; a married woman who is a bit on the plump side fears that her husband will be unfaithful with some dream creature, and the mistress (when she has a tendency to fat) is frightened of being left for a bright young thing of twenty with an insultingly perfect figure.

These women are sometimes only "fat" in their heads, blaming their excess weight for everything that is wrong in their lives. Whatever the case, the best thing is to do a serious assessment.

Some of the tables for calculating ideal weight which have been current in the last few years based on height are more or less useless. Some of them were too dogmatic and others not strict enough.

How can you calculate your ideal weight?

There are presently two approaches to calculating ideal weight, and these are now mentioned in most textbooks.

1. The Lorenz formula

$$\text{Ideal weight} = (\text{height in cm} - 100) - \frac{(\text{height} - 150)}{2}$$

Therefore, if you are 1 m 70 tall, you should weight sixty kilos, which seems about normal.

218

However, if you are 1 m 50 tall, your ideal weight will be fifty kilos, which seems a bit too much.

2. BMI (Body Mass Index) or the Quetelet formula

This is certainly the best there is. In any case it has now been internationally recognised.

It shows the ratio of weight (in kilos), divided by height (in metres and squared).

$$BMI = \frac{W}{H^2}$$

With the help of the above data, you can instantly calculate your BMI:

– With a BMI of 20 to 23: you are normal size
– With a BMI of 24 to 29: you are overweight
– With a BMI of over 30: we can speak of obesity.

Contrary to the Lorentz formula, this one has the advantage of giving you a wider spread of "normality" meaning that you do not have to concentrate on weight itself.

The fat map

The scales are paradoxically not the best tool to measure excess weight, as your weight is the sum of various masses: those of the skeleton, muscles, the veins, water and fat.

Obesity cannot only be defined as excess fat. In women the fat mass makes up about 25 % of body weight. A sportswoman may be slightly heavier, due to the her muscular mass, but it does not follow that she is fat.

On the other hand, water alone represents two thirds of body weight and may vary and easily lead to weight varia-

219

tions around one to two kilos, especially before and after menstruation.

This brings us to the conclusion that *"slimming"* and *"losing weight"* are two different things. Slimming means only losing excess fat, whereas weight may be lost purely by losing water, hence the futility – let alone the dangers – of diuretics which are often prescribed for slimming.

1. Measuring fat volume

There is now one way of measuring fat volume exactly, and this is the impedance meter. You are plugged into a machine (like an electrocardiogram), and you can see your water, muscle and fat masses written up on the screen.

This machine makes it possible to measure a person's fat volume and to keep track of it throughout the slimming phase. Unfortunately very few nutrition doctors are yet equipped with it.

In addition, these machines only identify the volume of the fat mass, without showing where it occurs in the body. This can however be done with a scanner, or even more easily be measuring the ratio of waist size (at the navel) to hip size. In any case, it should be less than 0.85. Let us now see what the various categories of obesity are.

2. Androidal obesity

If the ratio is too high, this is characteristic of androidal obesity, which prevails over the upper part of the body: face, neck, thorax, abdomen (above the navel).

We now know that extra weight of the androidal type can give a predisposition to some metabolic complications: diabetes, high blood pressure, hyperinsulinism, hypercholesterolemia, hypertriglyceridemia and heart diseases.

With this kind of obesity the fat cells (or adipocytes) are hypertrophied by an excess of fat, but usually their number remains stable.   In this case slimming will be relatively easy to achieve.

3. Gynoidal obesity

When the fat mass predominates mostly in the lower part of the body (lower abdomen, hips, thighs, buttocks), we can speak of gynoidal obesity.

When this is the case, the above-mentioned metabolic problems are rare, but there is often a weakness in the veins as well as knee and hip arthrosis.   The damage here can be as much mechanical as æsthetic.   This is often taken badly by the women concerned as it is very often associated with another disfigurement: cellulite.

4. Deep-seated fat deposits

A third kind of fat distribution has recently been identified. This is excess stomach fat around the blood vessels.   This deep fat deposit is often invisible from the "outside" as the waistline seems absolutely normal, but it is nevertheless dangerous as it carries a high risk of diabetes or cardio-vascular disease.

Women who smoke are especially at risk of having these deep fat deposits which are associated with normal weight.

Set yourself realistic objectives

Even if, as we have seen, your scales only give you a partial assessment of your weight, they are, even so, the tool which is most used to judge progress in slimming, based on the objective initially set.

But this objective must be realistic!   It would be Utopic

for a woman of fifty to want to go back her weight at twenty, especially as a good start is more likely if you begin slimming with some realistic hope of success rather than with the discouraging perspective of trying to achieve a mythical weight, come what may.

But the question that should also be asked before undertaking this slimming programme is that of knowing what you are really seeking by wishing to lose weight. Will you be able to cope with the new body image? Sometimes, taking a sudden interest in your weight may be symptomatic of another latent problem, such as family or marriage difficulties for example.

Latent problems are even more serious, however, as the need to slim is not always justified. Some women may thus be suffering from psychological troubles which losing weight may reveal. The opposite may be true for others, as the extra weight may be an unconscious barrier against the world, and often against men. Becoming once more a sexually desirable being then becomes insupportable.

It is obvious that in these circumstances it is very difficult to diagnose yourself. If you think seriously about it, you may question your motives. Anyway, even if all women do not necessarily need to slim, there has never been anything against wanting to correct bad nutritional habits, as far as I know! This is just what we were recommending in the first part of this book.

If you do not really feel up to undertaking PHASE I with the main aim of losing weight, just using the general principles of the Method (PHASE II) will be enough. This will enable you not only to change your body, and this will not come amiss as it will be a gradual process, but also to adopt a lifelong eating pattern which will be much richer nutritionally, and this can only have the effect of improving your physical health and improving your morale.

CHAPTER II

FOOD SYMBOLISM

Everyone knows that we live not from food alone, but that through the food that we eat we are also eating symbols. Eating refers back to the Mother, or at the very least to infancy, which means our upbringing. The way in which we eat also has a cultural dimension: national, regional or even religious.

There are however some women who have lost (or never known) this special relationship to food. They sit down to eat just as they would go to a garage to "fill up" the tank.

Very often, they do not even sit down. Morning coffee is drunk standing up with their coat already on, and at lunch time a sandwich or some kind of hamburger is gulped down in record time, on their own, elbows on a shelf, facing the wall in a fast food outlet.

This is how many of us have little by little lost any idea of "structure" and "socialising" at mealtimes, which has led to snacking at any time, like a dog which goes to its dish and eats biscuits when it feels the urge. Brillat-Savarin's famous aphorism *"animals nourish themselves, man eats and only a clever man knows how to eat"* has never been so true.

The lack of interest that people have in food, which has been reduced merely to its organic function, like in the

United States, can only lead to a veritable nutritional delinquency, which is at the root of excess weight and metabolic illnesses (diabetes, cardio-vascular diseases, etc.).

This then leaves the door open to de-structuring of eating patterns, stepping stones being most frequently eating snacks between meals and going without lunch, and then a huge dinner becomes the only real "meal" of the day.

A poll which appeared in ELLE in October 1991 showed that 15 % of French women consider that eating is a task and something they try to get over with as quickly as possible by hurrying the meal.

Comfort food

Bad food training often starts in the cradle. When a baby cries, the mother often correlates this to a distress or hunger signal. The baby may however just be "hungry" for a presence or for a cuddle. If it is calmed down by being given food every time it cries, when it grows up it will keep the same reflex. When it needs affection or love it will compensate with food.

Oral satisfaction, the first "sexual act" of a small baby, and an initiating stage in its psycho-affective development, will weigh heavily on its subsequent life, not only as regards food, but also in its relationships with others. The act of eating, even as an adult, can replace absent love, as if another person is not available, food is always there at hand.

The first little food behaviour difficulty is apparent therefore when small quantities of food are consumed repetitively without hunger as a motivation: this is snacking. The cigarette smoking habit is often a channel for this type of anxiety too.

The next stage is when the subject has sudden and irresistible impulses that lead her to eat a lot of a particular kind of food outside regular meal times, whether or not she is hungry. After the first pleasure, the subject also has a great feeling of guilt.

When the product is based on sugar, this sometimes leads to quite an addiction, as foods with sugar then correlate to childhood treats. Sugar is also a "pleasure food" eating of which may release endorphins into the body. This "internal morphine" which is secreted by the body itself will give a feeling of well-being.

At worst, food behavioural disturbances may lead to the appearance of an irresistible desire to eat: bulimia. Large amounts of food are then gulped down voraciously, in far greater quantities than are needed to satisfy hunger. This behaviour is so perverse that bulimic people do not hesitate to make themselves sick so that they don't get fat.

When some women realise that they are behaving abnormally they may be so self-deprecating that they slide into a state of depression, and through the see-saw effect, they then become anorexic, which is characterised by the disappearance of feelings of hunger and a very troubled relationship to food. Even when there is no previous history of psychiatric disorder, weight loss can become an obsession.

This obsession leads young anorexics (they are generally under twenty-five years old) to go down to less than forty kilos, which often necessitates being sent to hospital and sometimes even leads to intensive care units to avoid death, which is still too frequently the issue (10 % of cases).

But, even if some eating disorders may be brought on by bad behaviour learnt in infancy, they are also often the consequence of restrictions imposed in adulthood. Low calorie diets, which are always proposed to treat obesity, also lead to the appearance of psychological difficulties which lead to bulimia and anorexia.

The frustrations engendered effectively create an obsession about food and lead to perverse food rituals. The subject becomes irritable, has changing moods, and when she lets down her guard may "flip" and develop compulsive behaviour. This failure to be able to control food impulses lowers self-esteem and may lead to nervous breakdown.

Eating for pleasure: the food of civilisation

Contrary to comfort food, which is the response to frustration, eating for pleasure corresponds to the legitimate satisfaction of a duel need: the physiological, that of sustenance, and the psychological, hedonistic need – though it is difficult to separate the two.

The art of gastronomy is that of emphasising all the subtleties of flavour with the aim of giving maximum satisfaction to the sense of taste.

Through this refinement we have always sought to give full measure to food, thereby doting it with a very real cultural dimension which cannot be dissociated from the level of civilisation of a society.

Meals for humanity traditionally satisfy a ritual, and it is precisely through our relationship to food that we have since the beginning of time progressively become civilised.

Meals eaten in company, with members of the family or friends and the preliminary preparation for the gathering around food, even if it was only cooking it, have always been a mark of human evolution.

Ethnologists well know that the degree of sophistication of the meal, its ritual, is in proportion to the development of the civilisation in question.

In the bourgeois tradition, meals have always been considered as an important part of the day. They were a real ceremony that it was in very bad taste to upset.

In one of his stories, Maupassant tells of a fallen aristocrat, who, having retired to a wood-cutter's shack in the middle of the forest, nonetheless continues the ritual by

226

dressing for dinner every evening. And this merely out of respect for the sacred moment that meals always represented in his eyes.

Unfortunately, today there has been a break with tradition that can be analysed as a cultural regression.

Firstly, because traditional culinary knowledge is no longer transmitted from mother to daughter. Secondly, because women now work and meals are most often eaten away from home. And finally, when people do get home, the time given to preparation of meals is reduced to almost nothing, and they fall back on frozen, pre-packed dishes, cooked in a micro-wave.

The time spent on meals has been greatly tested by the development of leisure activities: television, video games, health clubs, etc. As meals are no longer considered to be an opportunity for social integration, the meal is more and more often considered to be a waste of time. This also explains why we do not spend more money than is strictly necessary on our food, and that is the minimum.

This progressive neglect of meals and food in general in our society though has contributed to the fact that the food/pleasure element has been forgotten in favour of practical and cheap snacking, and we are now rediscovering the nutritional dimension of the former.

It is in this climate of declining culinary and gastronomic values that the chaotic food behaviour patterns have developed, particularly in women, which we deplored previously. This is what is responsible for overweight, fatigue and many of the so-called illnesses of civilisation.

From this we can better understand how, in such a context, the fashion for meal substitutes (protein packets) has been able to develop: this now represents the main safety net for all those who hope to rid themselves of their surplus weight.

The need to rediscover food

Now you can see why you can never effectively undertake the application of the nutritional principles of this book if you have not previously rediscovered the role of and an interest in food, and more particularly in meals.

We have to undertake a veritable re-conquest of food, so that it is no longer seen as the enemy, but as a true friend. In order to discover, tame and master it more effectively, you only have to learn to love it. And who is better placed than a woman to understand that love and pleasure cannot be separated?

CHAPTER III

ADOLESCENCE

Adolescence is a very important stage in the life of a human being, and particularly for those of the female sex. It is effectively during this period that the body of a little girl metamorphosises completely due to the many organic upheavals as well as a really explosive hormonal change, to become that of a woman.

Knowing this we can well imagine the importance that food may assume.

This is why I am proposing firstly to run through the question in this chapter, by establishing something like a register of damage and then go on to an inventory of all the appropriate solutions and recommendations.

Stop nutritional delinquency!

All the polls on adolescent eating habits in France are worrying.

As far as quantity is concerned, energy input is more or less sufficient, as it is around 2 000 calories a day and only 7 % of adolescent girls eat a lot.

However, the distribution of this input throughout the day

leaves much to be desired. Statistics on breakfast, which only makes up 15 % of their food intake, are enlightening:

– 30 % say they are not hungry when they get up,
– 24 % say they do not have time to eat in the morning,
– 7 % never eat breakfast.

To conclude, more than 60 % of adolescent girls miss one of the main meals of the day, a practice which leads to increased liquid intake between meals and therefore often to eating between meals.

These snacks are mostly cakes or pastries, or salty delicacies and sweetened drinks. They are more rarely made up of fruit, and therefore constitute over-consumption of bad carbohydrates (white sugar and flour), saturated fats and salt, but above all foods which are nutritionally poor (lack of vitamins, mineral salts and oligo-elements).

The Val-de-Marne study, undertaken in 1988, gives a good idea of the magnitude of the deficit in micro-nutrient input, as a proportion of desirable amounts.

Here we can see large deficiencies in calcium, magnesium and vitamins, which are in fact particularly indispensable during this period when bodily transformations are very great.

MICRO-NUTRIENTS	GAP IN INPUT FOR ADOLESCENT GIRLS
Calcium	– 35 %
Magnesium	– 30 %
Iron	– 4 %
Zinc	– 29 %
Vitamin E	– 78 %
Vitamin B9	– 78 %
Vitamin B2	– 17 %
Vitamin B6	– 85 %
Vitamin B12	– 5 %
Vitamin C	– 2 %
Vitamin A	– 75 %

The results can be explained by the priority wrongly given to some foods to the detriment of others which are disliked to the point that some girls would not hesitate to call them "disgusting". These are, naturally, the foods which are of exceptional richness in micro-nutrients.

In 1990 a study made by the CREAS (the French Centre for Research on Children and Adolescents) showed that some foods were unknown to most girls: broccoli, rhubarb, water-cress, sorrel (to more than 50 % of them), split peas, pumpkin, celery and salsifi (to more than 30 %).

It was also found that:

– 15 % of young girls never eat fruit,
– 27 % never drink milk,
– 30 % never eat cheese.

On the other hand, they found that consumption of sweet drinks (processed fruit juices, Colas) was particularly high, which was as expected.

The study included much more interesting information that could enlighten us concerning the consumer habits of adolescent girls.

PREFERRED FOODS	FOODS WHICH ARE DISLIKED
Commercial fruit juices	Brains
Pancakes (*crêpes*)	Tripe
Pizza	Kidneys
Ice cream	Sweetbreads
Chips	Chitterlings (*andouilettes*)
Savoury tarts (quiche)	Liver
Danish pastries	Eggs
Cakes	Unpasteurised cheese
Mashed potato	Oysters
White pasta	Black pudding
Carrots	Wine
White ham	
Fruit yoghurt	
Red fruit	
(strawberries, cherries, raspberries)	

SWEET DRINKS	DAILY CONSUMPTION
• from 0 to 25 cl	52 %
• from 25 to 50 cl	23 %
• from 75 to 100 cl	10 %
• more than 100 cl	8 %
	7 %

AGE GROUPS	% OF ADOLESCENT GIRLS WHO SMOKE
• from 10-11 years	5.5 %
• from 12-13 years	7.5 %
• from 14-15 years	21.5 %
• from 16-17 years	42.5 %
• from 18-24 years	65.5 %

Consumption of alcoholic beverages amongst girls of sixteen:

– 56 % regularly drink spirits (10 % of them several times a week);
– 25 % regularly drink beer (an average of 1 litre a week);
– 21 % regularly drink wine (an average of 50 cl a week).

Other studies have led us to conclude that:

– 33 % of adolescent girls have already been drunk once before they were sixteen (45 % in vocational secondary schools, and 17 % in other secondary schools);
– 22 % of them "get high" on alcohol more than ten times a year, especially in the less affluent classes.

Smoking, which is characteristic of adolescence, is no less alarming:

At sixteen, the percentage of girls who smoke more than twelve cigarettes a day was:

– lower sixth form..................... 17 %
– upper sixth form .... 30 %

– vocational sixth form............ 48 %
– work release courses............ 61 %

Nowadays adolescent girls who give priority to their studies are usually treated like boys and do not have to do any housework. It naturally follows that they frequently do not know much about cooking, as the techniques and culture of cooking are not transmitted to them by their mothers. More than 30 % of them cannot even cook an egg!

This break with tradition has emerged from a certain lack of interest in meals, their preparation, and as a consequence, in gastronomy in general.

It will be understood in this context that ready prepared dishes or fast food may be the best answer to the need to feed oneself.

The meal, which has completely lost its happy convivial dimension, is no longer the setting for precious conversation that is used to be. In addition if you ask adolescent girls what activity they prefer when they want to enjoy themselves, they reply:

– 28 %, go to the cinema
– 24 %, listen to music
– 19 %, sports
– 17 %, discussion
– 11 %, reading
– and only 6 % chose sharing a good meal.

For an education in "good eating"

Given the sad state of affairs that we have just described, the first thing to be done is to make adolescent girls aware of the importance of their way of eating for their present and future health.

Contrary to what some may believe, the body of an adolescent girl, even if it is already formed, has not yet reached the stage of maturity. It is not yet "adult". It therefore needs adequate food to finish its growth. In addition, not only her present physical and intellectual well-being depend on proper food, but also her future state of health.

Here is some general advice that I would like to give them.

1. Have sufficient protein intake

This can be calculated at a rate of 1.2 grams per kilo of weight and can be obtained from meat, fish, eggs and cheese, and also from vegetable proteins (Soya, pulses, whole foods, cereals, nuts).

2. Make sure you have enough calcium

This implies having milk products or cheese at every meal.

This calcium input will enable you not only to complete construction of the skeleton, but also ensure prevention of risk of bone deficiency during future pregnancy and above all after menopause (osteoporosis and fractures). A daily intake of 1 200 mg of calcium is necessary.

For more information, you will find below a list of foods which, in the quantities given, will provide 300 mg of calcium. You only need to eat four portions of these in a day, or even eat them together.

FOODS RICH IN CALCIUM (300 MG PER PORTION)	
30 grams of gruyère cheese 50 grams of camembert 2 yoghurts 1/4 litre milk (about half a pint) 300 grams of *fromage blanc* 10 small individual cream cheeses *(petits-suisses)*	100 grams semolina 150 grams water cress 150 grams almonds or hazelnuts 400 grams wholemeal bread 850 grams green cabbage 4 large oranges 1 kilo fish 2 kilo meat

3. Have sufficient iron intake

We have seen that an iron deficiency is one of the most serious for an adolescent girl.

Such neglect of foods containing iron (see the table above) occurs at a time when needs for iron are increased by tissue growth in her body and the increase of red blood corpuscles.

Also, at menstruation time, a loss of iron occurs which is even greater when blood loss is longer and more abundant.

It has to be recognised that lack of iron leads to anaemia and fatigue, a lowering of physical and intellectual performance as well as lower resistance to infection.

Lack of iron may even seriously impede slimming as it helps the natural production of L-Carnitine, an enzyme which speeds the use free fatty acids.

The necessary daily iron ration for a young girl is 18 mg, but two kinds can be mentioned:

– heminic iron, which comes from meat and fish and of which 25 % is absorbed;
– non-heminic iron, found in vegetables and of which only 5 % is absorbed.

This shows how difficult it is for vegetarians to have sufficient iron intake.

SOURCES OF HEMINIC IRON (PER 100 GRAMS)		SOURCES OF NON-HEMINIC IRON (PER 100 GRAMS)	
Clams (seafood)	25 mg	Pure Cocoa powder	15 mg
Mussels	25 mg	70 % cacao chocolate	10 mg
Black sausage	20 mg	Broad beans	10 mg
Pork liver	15 mg	Haricot beans	8 mg
Beef of lamb liver	10 mg	Lentils	7 mg
Egg yoke	7 mg	Nuts	5 mg
Oysters	6 mg	Dry fruit	4 mg
Calf liver	5 mg	Spinach	4 mg
Meat	3 mg	Wholemeal bread	3 mg
Poultry and fish	2 mg		

Finally, it must be stated that a diet rich in tannins (wine, tea) and fibres can somewhat limit the absorption of iron.

4. Have an optimum vitamin intake

For this you must absolutely avoid processed foods and choose whole cereals as well as pulses (lentils, dry beans, chick peas, etc.).

Supplements of dry yeast and wheat germ, such as we recommend, are almost indispensable for an adolescent girl.

She should also, as we have mentioned elsewhere, eat fruit and raw vegetables every day (rich in vitamin C) and give preference to foods which are rich in vitamin E: olive oil, sunflower oil, nuts, etc.

Slimming for Adolescent Girls

In the old days girls around eleven years old, before their first communion, were slim, frail or even thin. From then on, the time of puberty, together with its hormonal changes, made them fill out a bit. Some of them even became rather plump and their faces were adorned with a few pimples.

At seventeen everything more or less went back to normal. Young girls certainly filled out (but only, thank goodness, to an extent corresponding to indispensable female attributes), but their figures became svelte once again.

At eighteen, their bodies reached their physical peak and their wasp waist emphasised the curve of their firm, high breasts, as did a well muscled posterior. It was the age of seduction, of love, and conventionally, that of marriage.

Today, modern little girls are often a little "rounded" before puberty. And there is nothing really surprising in this as beginning with infant foods made of flour, her daily food has been made up of nothing but ravioli and white rice, potatoes, frozen stuffed pancakes, quiches and pizzas, not forgetting the famous sweets, biscuits, snack bars and highly sweetened fizzy drinks. From infancy onwards therefore, her pancreas has been sorely tried.

The onset of adolescence, with the hormonal upsets of which we are aware, is therefore even more of a handicap because eating habits deteriorate further: fast food, Coke pastry snacks and alcoholic beverages.

She quickly puts on pounds. To counterbalance this, she will miss meals and blindly enter upon low calorie diets the consequences of which (described in the first part of this book) are even more accentuated because the body is particularly sensitive as it is in the middle of changes.

The consequences of these diets are quite classical:

- increase in fat cells (hyperplasia) because of the restrictions. The body is even more inclined to this as it is undergoing complete change;
- aggravation of lacks of nutrients which may lead to serious health problems: fatigue, anaemia, sensitivity to infections;
- return to higher weight through the rebound effect phenomenon with fatal risks for the subject's morale;
- development of classic food behavioural problems: bulimia then anorexia.

Bulimia and anorexia

Apparently opposites, these two behavioural problems in fact alternate in adolescent girls. A young girl begins by developing what specialists call a "dysmorphophobia", which means a bad self-image (35 % of them do not like their body). This rejection of her own appearance leads her to want to emulate fashionable standards of slimness and voluntarily choose to restrict her food intake. This is the anorexic phase.

Then, as she is hungry and this hunger becomes insup-

237

portable, she begins compulsive eating. This is the bulimia phase, which may be accompanied by self-inflicted vomiting or even taking of laxatives, diuretics or appetite depressors, as we mentioned earlier.

This situation is particularly dangerous as she is then likely to cause a lowering in the potassium level which can be responsible for cardiac rhythm difficulties and intense muscular fatigue. These eating behavioural problems are much more frequent outside France (especially in the Anglo-Saxon countries) where there are virtually no cultural factors related to feeding. In France, according to the statistics, periods of bulimia are still found in 6 % of girl students and anorexia in 3 to 4 % of adolescent girls.

Even though behavioural treatments manage to improve considerably the fate of those suffering from bulimia, forecasts for anorexics on the other hand are less optimistic, in spite of oft repeated hospital stays.

A "highway code" for slimmers

It is recognised that women are capable of great determination, and this is just one of their qualities. One of their failings though is that they do not always see the nuances, which sometimes leads them to excessive behaviour. But, as far as food is concerned, a happy mean should always be respected.

The general advice in Part I of this book is valid for everyone. I do think however, that it is not necessary for an adolescent girl undertake an accelerated slimming phase such as that in Phase I.

Apart from pathological obesity, which needs specialist guidance (an endocrinologist for example), a few extra pounds may disappear for good with just a simple readjustment of eating habits (Phase II).

In any case, adolescent girls should read the whole of the first part of the book. It is in effect important that they understand both how their body works and how to recognise foods in order to be able to choose them wisely. It is no use going without one food or another on the excuse that it is fattening. What has to be realised is that no food, taken individually, is fattening – neither butter nor potatoes. It is the interaction of foods amongst themselves and the triggering of particular of metabolic mechanisms by certain foods that may lead to weight gain.

This being said, here is a list of advice which should suffice for an adolescent girl to recover her normal weight balance and a greater vitality.

– Eat three meals a day and be careful to never miss one of them.

– Avoid high glycaemic index carbohydrates and notably those with a very high index: potatoes, white flours, sugar, etc.

– Avoid eating between meals. If you feel a bit peckish in the middle of the day, you can either eat fruit, including dried fruit (especially figs), or, at teatime, for example, eat a slice of wholemeal bread with 100 % fruit, unsweetened marmalade. You can also treat yourself from time to time to something sweet: a few squares of 70 % (or more) cacao chocolate.

– Avoid fast food outlets for your main meals. If you go to a pizzeria, order the aubergines with cheese or tomato with mozzarella. If you have to, it would be better to eat white pasta, which has a glycaemic index of 55/60 rather than things which have been made with white flour (pizza, hamburgers, hot-dogs, etc.), or chips, even though they have one of the highest glycaemic indexes.

– Rediscover your grandmother's recipes: salt pork with lentils *(petit salé aux lentilles)*, dried beans, split peas, beef stew with turnips, cabbage and leeks.

– Eat milk products. Have skimmed milk in the morning for breakfast. Eat cheese. Rediscover the wealth of local

239

produce. If you do not like cheese, then eat yoghurt, as much as you like.

– For breakfast, have wholemeal bread on which you can put a little butter, or try raw cereals or even muesli. They are good, practical and quick to prepare.

– Do not give up fat altogether, rather choose good fats, those from fish (herring, salmon, mackerel, sardines), olive, walnut and sunflower oil.

– Cut out all processed drinks, and especially Coke. Instead, have freshly squeezed fruits with no added sugar. Allow yourself a glass of red wine from time to time, for example at the end of a weekend meal. If you are offered an aperitif, never have spirits. Ask rather for a tomato juice, or sometimes for a glass of wine.

– Rediscover the pleasure of eating and cooking. Do not believe as your mothers did for a time that it is degrading to spend time cooking nice little recipes. Cooking is, on the contrary, an art in itself. These days, a "Chef" has more prestige than an computer programmer.

Does the pill make you fat?

Nearly 70 % of adolescent girls between eighteen and twenty-one take the pill. But pharmaceutical companies remain strangely silent on the subject of the possible effects of the anti-conception pill on the weight of its users.

In the past, it was difficult to refute the fact that the first generations of pills caused weight gain. It is almost certain now that third generation pills, which are those in use today, have no weight implications, or at least not for adolescent girls who are already slim.

At most a gain of about two kilos can be noticed sometimes in the first six months. This latter does not necessarily correspond, however, to an increased fat accumulation, but rather to additional water retention due to taking oestrogens.

When weight gain occurs later than this, it would seem to be rather an excess of fat due to the anabolic effects of progesterone.

Scientific data available on this subject shows, however, that there is a risk of excessive secretion of insulin even with the third generation pills.

It would therefore seem that for women who are already subject to hyperinsulinism, insulin resistance and in addition have a weight problem (obesity) the pill can only lead to more metabolic problems.

This is even more likely as doctors do not necessarily automatically prescribe third generation pills, with less secondary effects, but continue to give second generation pills to their patients.

To sum up, be on your guard, and this applies even more to adolescent girls who are starting the pill when they are already over weight. According to individual sensitivity, weight gain cannot be excluded. Above three kilos, it would be advisable to bring it to the attention of the doctor who prescribed it.

Respect of the principles of the Method is even more advisable in this case, as they are precisely designed to reduce hyperinsulinemia.

On the other hand, it must be recognised that the pill generally improves acne and that some of them have even been specially adapted for this purpose.

Adolescence, sport and nutrition

For an adolescent girl it is not only preferable to do physical exercise, but highly recommended. Doing a sport regularly and in moderation, is a guarantee of good health for the muscle, respiratory and cardiac systems, without mentioning that it is certainly the best means of enjoying yourself with your friends, girls and boys.

As the protein ration for a sportswoman whose body is developing should be quite high (1.5 grams per kilo of weight per day), she should see that her meat, fish, milk product and egg consumption is increased, and at the same time drink a lot of water so as to eliminate uric acid and urea due to the effort.

Muscles are naturally the organs upon which the most demand is made when doing a sporting activity. Their main fuel is, as you know, glucose. But, this glucose is stored in the body in the form of glycogen (in the liver and muscle tissues which are somewhat like reservoirs). After digestion all the carbohydrates are transformed into glucose (except for fructose).

For a long time sports people were advised to eat "slow carbohydrates" to take account of the physical effort. We now know that this idea was wrong and that before any muscular effort it is low glycaemic index carbohydrates that should be eaten (fruit, cereals, wholemeal bread, pulses, whole pasta).

Eating potatoes, white rice, sweets and cakes can only lead to a rapid rise in glycaemia (increase of glucose in the blood), the consequence of which will be, as we know, an increased secretion of insulin.

This could be the cause of severe hypoglycaemia, two or three hours after eating, the main characteristic of which will be the appearance of fatigue which will restrict the physical activity – a sudden feeling of being drained.

The day before an important sports event, the following programme is advisable:

– have a dinner built around low glycaemic index car-bohydrates such as wholemeal pasta or pulses (lentils, beans, chick peas, wholemeal semolina, etc.). This input of good carbohydrates is what will enable you to sustain an effort over a longer period;

– for breakfast, which should if possible be eaten three hours before the sporting activity, you should have whole-meal bread together with unsweetened jam or marmalade and/or whole cereals (without sugar), with a 0 % fat milk product (hot or cold milk, yoghurt or *fromage blanc*);

Supplementary information

– Alcohol is a fuel that the muscles do not know how to use. Contrary to some preconceived notions it cannot therefore help muscular effort in any way. This is especially true of beer. In addition, alcoholic beverages being diuretics, they have the effect of aggravating dehydration.

– The Scandinavian diet consisting of going without carbohydrates from the sixth to the fourth day before a sporting competition, and then to only eat pasta and rice for the three days before the test, must be reserved for very high level sports people under strict medical supervision. This is not adapted to amateur sports.

– Muscle cramp and stitch can be caused by several things: insufficient hydration, lack of glycogen, hypoglycaemic state, an excess of acid in the muscles, etc.

– As sports require a lot of water, especially if it is hot, the sports person must drink often, having small mouthfuls of water with lemon juice or tea from the time they awake. It is well known that lack of hydration is very frequent amongst sportsmen and women;

– while you are exerting yourself, especially over a long period, you should have a continuous supply of glycogen so as to avoid suddenly running out.

– When you have to make a particularly great muscular effort, insulin secretion is automatically low, even insignificant. Drinking regularly when doing a sport is not only advisable but necessary. For this, you should have already prepared a litre of water, mixed with four soup spoons of fructose and the juice of two lemons.

If the sport permits (bicycle), you can eat as many dry fruits or energy providing bars as you like (raw cereal bars, marzipan or fruit bars).

In this way, thanks to well planned eating and with minimal muscle and breathing training, your few hours, or even your day of sporting activity will take place in the best physical conditions, without sudden tiredness or excessive fatigue.

Like this, sport will become a real source of pleasure for an adolescent girl.

How to have a nice skin

The condition of skin, hair and nails often reflects the state of health. A dull skin, greasy broken or split hair, nails with white blotches or which split, show there is something wrong. The cause of these troubles is often to be found in a badly balanced diet, which leads to vitamin, oligo-element, mineral salt, sulphated amino acid and essential fatty acid deficiency.

In fact, vitamins A and E are essential to the quality of the skin [1].

– Vitamin B5 aids skin hydration and fortifies the hair follicles;
– Vitamin B8 prevents hair becoming greasy or falling out;
– Zinc regulates secretion of sebum (which is abnormal in the case of acne) and contributes to good hair condition.

---

1. See the table of vitamins in Chapter VI, Part. I.

These micro-nutrients can of course be found in various cosmetic products that are used daily, but the more certain way of obtaining them is by keeping to a nutritionally rich diet.

Taking synthetic food supplements, which are not well absorbed by the intestine, is not a good solution. On the other hand, your food can be supplemented by two natural products which are particularly rich in nutrients: wheat germ and brewer's yeast.

Acne, which appears around puberty, is due to an excess of sebum (the oily secretion of the skin) and is complicated by inflammation and infection.

This therefore has no relationship to food. "Spotty" adolescent girls can therefore continue to eat chocolate (over 70 % cacao content) and salami *(saucisson)* without having to worry. Overdoing things, lack of sleep and smoking can, however, seriously contribute to deterioration of the skin.

How to prevent cellulite

Cellulite puts adult women to shame, as it is during this period of her existence that it is the most obvious. It is however the result of a long process which begins in adolescence. The best way of avoiding it is therefore to prevent it.

Cellulite is caused by many factors: genetic, hormonal, circulation, food and psychological, but the initial factor is always hormones. It is due to an excess secretion of, or over-sensitivity to oestrogens, even when they are present in normal quantities. The latter act upon the fat cells (or adipocytes) by helping their growth in number or in size.

This bloating of the fat cells will happen even more readily if the fat distribution of the subject is of the gynoidal type (tendency to larger buttocks, hips and thighs).

The way in which cellulite occurs is simple: through the action of oestrogens, the adipocytes (fat cells gorged with fat) increase in volume and constrict the blood vessels. The circulation is then impaired.

The sub-cutaneous layer thickens (hence the famous orange peel effect), cell waste is badly evacuated and water movement perturbed and the nerve fibres are constricted (causing pain).

The supporting conjunctive tissue hardens and ends by separating the fat deposits. Amongst the hormones which are partially responsible for cellulite are insulin (high secretion of which is caused by the wrong foods, as we have seen from the beginning of this book).

In case of stress, the corticoids of the surrenal glands also come into the picture and can lead to cellulite development.

The first preventive measure naturally consists in avoiding all nutritional delinquency by applying the nutritional principles contained in this book.

If the subject already has leg circulation problems with a tendency to swelling after puberty, then hot baths should be avoided as also should too long exposure to sun. A treatment directed towards fighting weakness in the veins could possibly be prescribed by your general practitioner.

It will also be necessary to avoid clothes and underclothes which are too tight, and which interfere with blood circulation (jeans and some tights).

Practising a sport will be necessary to fight the bad effects of a sedentary lifestyle, especially as insufficiently developed muscles leave room for the development of fatty areas.

Finally, it is never too early to learn to manage stress. Techniques like yoga and sophrology are very helpful for this.

CHAPTER IV

A WOMAN OF THIRTY

An adult woman, of which the woman of thirty is the archetype, is by very definition in her prime. Adolescence is only a vague memory and menopause, the idea of which is almost inconceivable, is a far horizon

This period in the life of a woman is generally marked by intense professional and sexual activity in a partnership or marriage, and pregnancy is the major event of consequence.

In this age group, spanning the ages from thirty to forty-five, women have varied eating habits. These differ according to upbringing, but above all depend on the time available to prepare meals.

Polls on eating habits show that these habits, even though they are better than those of adolescent girls, are generally such that they eventually lead to weakening the body.

The studies have shown that excesses (too much sugar, too much salt, too much white flour) and insufficiencies (not enough vegetables or milk products or liquids) may expose women to deficiencies (iron, vitamin C, E, B, calcium and magnesium deficiencies). Added to this there is a real risk of weight gain and cellulite, without mentioning chronic fatigue. Readjusting eating habits is therefore particularly necessary for this category of women, as they would like to be not only attractive, but also absolutely fit.

The fitness programme

The advice we gave in the chapter on adolescence remains valid here with, however, a few nuances. In order to avoid fatigue and high vulnerability to stress, attention should be focused on some specific points.

1. Ensure a sufficient magnesium intake

The modern tendency consisting of giving precedence to processed foods to the detriment of natural, and raw foods such as pulses, leads to a chronic deficiency in magnesium. French women usually have a daily intake of 210 mg of magnesium, whilst the recommended dose is 330 mg. This

MAGNESIUM CONTENT			
PROCESSED FOODS (PAR 100 GRAMS)		**RAW FOODS** (PER 100 GRAMS)	
White bread	30 mg	Wholemeal bread	80 mg
White rice	30 mg	Brown rice	140 mg
White pasta	52 mg	Wholemeal pasta	70 mg

FOODS RICH IN MAGNESIUM	
Cocoa powder (van Houten)	420 mg/100 g
Wheat germ	400 mg/100 g
Almonds	260 mg/100 g
70 % cacao chocolate	260 mg/100 g
Dried beans	160 mg/100 g
Walnuts and hazelnuts	140 mg/100 g
Brown rice	140 mg/100 g
Oat flakes	130 mg/100 g
Lentils	90 mg/100 g
Wholemeal bread	90 mg/100 g
Dried figs	85 mg/100 g
Wholemeal pasta	70 mg/100 g

deficiency can lead to fatigue, cramps, hyper-emotivity and "spasmophilia".

2. Having enough Vitamin B6

Tiredness, coupled with irritability, and even a bit of depression in women on the pill, are usually due to a vitamin B6 deficiency. The Val-de-Marne study shows that 85 % of women have an intake below the recommended amount because of bad eating habits. This deficiency may be aggravated by taking the pill, recent motherhood or over consumption of glutamates.

We know also that insufficient vitamin B, in addition to the symptoms already mentioned, can lead to feelings of dizziness, upset sebum secretion (greasy skin and hair), and also to a strong desire for sugary things (because of lack of serotonin).

The recommended dose of vitamin B6 is 2 mg a day. This may be obtained from the following foods:
- brewer's yeast .... 4 mg per 100 g
- wheat germ .... 3 mg per 100 g
- bean sprouts................. 1.5 mg per 100 g
- avocado .... 0.60 mg per 100 g
- pulses......................... 0.50 mg per 100 g
- brown rice .... 0.50 mg per 100 g
- fish............................. 0.40 mg per 100 g

3. Having enough Vitamin C

Even if the debate amongst experts which is taking place at the moment about whether or not Vitamin C (in large doses) has tonic effects, no conclusion has yet been reached, and we are now convinced that many of its effects are quite beneficial:

- it stimulates the body's defences against infection
- it helps to fight against stress by aiding the synthesis of certain hormones (steroids)
- it helps to absorb iron and synthesise L-Carnitine;
- it protects against the bad effects of cigarette smoke.

And the opposite is true of a lack of vitamin C which can cause some problems:

– fatigue;
– loss of breath when making an effort;
– drowsiness;
– muscle aches;
– risks of infection.

This is why a daily intake of between 80 – 90 mg of vitamin C is recommended.

For a woman who smokes, the need for vitamin C is particularly high. It is known in fact that smoking a packet of cigarettes a day destroys about 50 mg of vitamin C.

Women smokers should therefore make sure that they have from 150 to 200 mg, according to how much they smoke, in order to avoid any deficiency and to protect their cells from oxidation.

It is useless and dangerous though to have too high an intake as this may lead to the appearance of stones in the urine (urinary pain).

Finally it must be said that synthetic vitamin C, which comes in pills, is not absorbed as well by the body as that contained naturally in foods.

FOODS CONTAINING 50 MG OF VITAMIN C	
30 g of black currents	70 g of water cress
25 g of kiwis	80 g of uncooked red cabbage
50 g of raw peppers	100 g of citrus fruits
25 g of parsley	200 g of liver or kidneys

4. Avoid any risk of hypoglycaemia

(Please refer to Chapter VI, Part I.)

Things which slow down slimming

As far as slimming is concerned, sexual equality is not always the rule. Even if a man and a woman eat all their meals together and have exactly the same food in quantity and in kind (in conformity with the principles of the Method), they may obtain completely different results. After a few months the man may be patting himself on the back for having, for example, lost ten kilos whilst the woman is moaning that she has only lost three.

Madam will then be tempted to think that *"the Montignac method works better for men than for women"*, forgetting rather quickly that her best friend (the one who advised her to buy the book) lost her eight kilos with no difficulty in only two months. Her conclusion will therefore have been a little hasty. It is in fact wrong to see the question in these terms, by trying to compare the incomparable. This is not only because the two women may have very different reactions, but also because the number of ways in which men and women differ is considerable.

1. Are women "fatter" than men?

The female body has a greater fatty mass than that of her male counterpart: 22 to 25 % as against 17 % for men. This "honour" is manifest in a greater number of fatty cells (adipocytes).

2. Fat is differently distributed

For a woman, the distribution of the fat mass is most often of the gynoidal type (below the waist), with the possible complication of cellulite. For men, it is more of the androidal type (above the waist).

This particular female topography (generous hips, buttocks and thighs) has a very specific natural function: that of ensuring an energy reserve for a possible pregnancy and milk production. The vital reason for this was to ensure sufficient reserves in case of famine or shortages of food, but this is an anachronism today in industrialised societies, but the female body often still retains the ancestral reflex.

The fatty cells in the lower body of a woman actually have special receivers which are "programmed" more specifically to accumulate reserves than to permit their release. Possible excess weight around this part of the anatomy is therefore more resistant to any attempt to slim.

3. Greater sensitivity to hormones

Contrary to man, woman, when she is sexually active, follows the rhythm of her hormones. Puberty, pregnancy, an oestrogen/progesterone imbalance and menopause, all these stages are risk factors which may possibly encourage weight gain.

During the pre-menstrual period, that is to say during the few days before a period, appetite may increase as well as a tendency to compulsive carbohydrate behaviour, i.e. a desire for sweet foods.

At this time there may also be a small tendency to depression (lowering of serotonin), and the desire for sugar can be explained more readily because it is precisely sugar which contributes to raising the level of serontonin.

It must be pointed out that some hormone treatments, when they are badly conducted, may also lead to weight gain (see Chapter V, Part I).

4. A woman with a past – one diet after another

Men generally start their first slimming diet between thirty-five and forty-five years old, when they come to do a radical stocktaking, and at the same time take up sports again, stop smoking, change their job, and even sometimes their wife. They may be said to be "diet virgins". Their body reacts much better and slimming goes more smoothly.

Women, on the other hand, will more readily go without some foods, and will start to do so even from puberty. They start the battle with the idea of fighting against a little plumpness due to adolescence, but also against hypothetical weight problems which are the consequence of the skeletal standards current in women's magazines.

Years pass like this, punctuated by constantly repeated low calorie diets. As time goes by, their bodies are weary of these successive weight losses, which are always followed by further increase, and their survival instinct sets off certain regulatory mechanisms, the aim of which is to regain the lost weight and above all to consolidate it, thus creating a resistance to any subsequent attempt to slim.

In order to achieve this, their bodies often even go as far as to increase the number of fat cells so as to be able to accumulate a maximum of reserves. And this is how obesity hypertrophies (the adipocytes are gorged with fat) and then becomes hyperplasic (new adipocytes are created).

5. Watch out for protein deficiencies!

Contrary to men, women are not very keen on meat. And in addition, they eat a lot less cheese and are easily put off by eggs. So, these likes and dislikes mean that their protein ration is often insufficient and leads to deficiencies when they undertake low calorie diets.

It has been clearly shown, though, that a nutritional deficiency in proteins prevents diminution of fat mass and brings about a kind of resistance to slimming.

6. The impact of stress

After serious emotional upsets (bereavement, divorce, unemployment, etc.), a woman will sometimes begin to lose weight. This is in fact only an automatic response to a forced diet.

She can't swallow anything because the stomach is "in knots" but this situation is generally only temporary. Faced with stress, the rule is more often an immediate or subsequent increase in weight.

If this happens, two groups of factors are the cause: behavioural factors and biochemical factors.

Behavioural factors

Faced with "feeling bad", oral reflexes take over and you eat to fill the void which is creating anxiety.

These behavioural eating problems show up, as we already said earlier, in various attitudes:

– systematic eating between meals;
– compulsive sugar eating, with or without "addiction";
– tendencies to bulimia, or overeating.

It has been seen that 40 % of women admit eating when they are fed up.

Biological factors

Stress triggers many biochemical reactions in the body:

– fall in the growth hormone;
– secretion of endorphins;
– secretion of cortisol.

These modifications stimulate lipogenesis, that is the storage of fats (directly or through the setting off hyperinsulinism).

Women are even more subject to this possible weight gain

than men. Their nutritional deficiencies (magnesium, vitamin B6, iron, etc.) make them more vulnerable.

Readjusting eating habits and enriching them nutritionally will enable you to naturally lower many of the risks of stress.

Eat well for nine months

Bearing a child is one of the most important experiences in the life of a woman, and this is why it is advisable for her to prepare for it mentally as well as physically.

If weight loss is necessary it should always take place before the pregnancy. Most women think, however, that because they are going to put on a bit of weight during the gestation period anyway there will be time enough afterwards to kill two birds with one stone. This is a mistake! If you are already overweight it is more than recommended that you should, as far as possible, lose weight before pregnancy, and this is so that you can avoid it setting in after the birth, but also, and even more so as to avoid foetal or maternal complications (high blood pressure, diabetes, eclampsia).

Losing weight using the usual low calorie principles would be particularly dangerous, as we know that this creates great deficiencies in vitamins, mineral salts and oligo-elements at a time when the human body needs them twice as much.

Only a diet undertaken in accordance with the recommendations of the Montignac Method can guarantee an intake of the nutrients indispensable for the correct development of the baby, as well as lasting results.

For nine months, the future mother must ensure the optimal development of the foetus without at the same time running out of her own reserves. This is why her food should be chosen in such a way as to give her the necessary

255

nutrients and spread them harmoniously over the whole day.

The general nutritional choices that we recommend will meet this need. We can add the following advice to the general principles.

– eating for two is unnecessary. However, you must make yourself to eat twice as well;

– make sure that you get enough animal proteins (meat, poultry, fish, eggs, milk products, etc.) and also vegetable proteins (whole foods, pulses, soya derivatives). Proteins effectively ensure the "construction" of the baby. You must though avoid eating liver more than once a week, so as to avoid any possible risk of vitamin A poisoning. You must also avoid uncooked meat, such as steak tatare, and also seafood (risk of infection);

– stock up on calcium, both to construct the child's skeleton but also to protect the mother's stocks. You should therefore eat a milk product at every meal (milk, cheese, yoghurt, *fromage blanc*);

– ensure that you receive enough fluoride, i.e. drinking mineral water which contains it (Badoit, Vichy);

– guarantee enough iron intake so as to avoid any possible anaemia, fatigue or vulnerability to infection (black pudding, meat, pulses, dried fruit and eggs);

– avoid any folic acid deficiency, which could lead to foetal malformation. To do this you should eat brewer's yeast, wheat germ and pulses:

– make sure you get enough fibres, not only because the foods that contain them are rich in vitamins and mineral salts, but also to avoid any risk of constipation. You must therefore regularly eat fruit, raw vegetables, green vegetables, salads, wholemeal bread and cereals and pulses;

– drink enough water to avoid dehydration, help passage through the intestines and avoid urinary infections.

Naturally, alcohol is to be avoided, as it is dangerous for the baby and you should only allow yourself, at the most, half a glass of red wine at the end of each meal. Polyphenols in alcohol contribute to improvement of the circulation;

– avoid, unless you have sought medical advice, taking medicines or dietary supplements;

– eat a variety of things so as to avoid any deficiencies, but also to get the child used to a certain dietary variety. From the fourth month of pregnancy, the foetus can notice tastes. The more foods that he has tasted in his mother's womb, the easier will be the diversification of his food upon weaning;

– finally, do not smoke as smoking can lead to a small baby.

During some pregnancies, a large weight gain is apparent (fifteen to twenty kilos) and this can never be justified. Normal weight gain is around eight kilos and can be broken down in the following way:

– 3.5 kilos for the foetus itself at birth;
– 500 g for the placenta;
– 1 kilo for the uterus;
– 700 g for the amniotic liquid;
– 1 kilo for the increased volume of the breasts;
– 1.3 kilos for the increase in the amount of blood.

The difference between the theoretical amount of weight gain (eight kilos) and a higher real gain can be explained in the following way: in the second term of pregnancy, the foetus does not get much bigger, but the mother may have a tendency (through an unconscious reflex) to naturally build up reserve fats in case a famine should occur at the end of the pregnancy. The risk of added weight is even greater if her food is hyperglycaemic (rich in bad carbohydrates). Following the principles of the Method will therefore be the best preventive measure.

Weight gain can also be linked to excessive water retention, with bruising sometimes, usually due to vein problems. In this case, strict medical supervision is imperative, as this situation may be a symptom of high blood pressure or albumin in the urine.

Whatever the cause, weight gain must be judged on the basis of the original starting weight, taking into account height. A woman weighing sixty kilos before her pregnancy and who is 1 m 50 tall must not put on more than eight kilos.

One who weighs fifty-two kilos and is 1 m 75 tall can gain fifteen kilos easily, as she is starting off with very low reserves. She will lose the extra very easily after the birth. Breast feeding also helps lose excessive fat. It is rather as though the body pumps out the reserves that it has built up. Breast feeding therefore helps you get your figure back.

The ubiquitous cellulite

Cellulite is something of a nightmare for all women, but unfortunately it only becomes a real worry when it has set in visibly.

This subject was already partially dealt with in the chapter on adolescence, but we can never overemphasise that the best way to get rid of this disfigurement is to prevent it as early as possible, well before you have seen the first symptoms.

It is however never too late to act, especially as it must

be admitted that there is not one solution, but a number of measures which, undertaken together, can seriously help to improve the situation.

Cellulite is the result of three factors:

- a natural predisposition in women;
- hormonal imbalance;
- bad eating habits;
- bad lifestyle.

By working on the last two factors, you can stop the development process, or even reverse it. But, once again, to manage this, you must tackle the overall problem, which implies revising your lifestyle. Here are a set of measures that you should take:

- Correct any excess weight

Reserve fats effectively aggravate vein compression due to cellulite. Once the excess weight has disappeared, it is easier to see what is really down to cellulite, especially as concerns the bad æsthetic aspect. It is then that one can, amongst other things, undertake possible localised treatment.

- Adopt good eating habits

This principle implies firstly giving up all bad eating habits. For this it will suffice to adopt the main principles of the Method[1] on a lifelong basis, which entails eating carbohydrates with a low glycaemic index rather than bad carbohydrates (with a high glycaemic index).

- Treat weak veins

Weak veins, more commonly known as "bad circulation" are an affliction which is common to women in general and

---

1. See Part I.

quite usual in those who show symptoms of cellulite. The circulatory problems to which it leads are made worse not only by a sedentary lifestyle but also by modern living habits: wearing clothes which are too tight, overheated baths, long exposure to the sun.

In the most serious cases, medical treatment can be of great help, but sometimes the old remedies used by our grandmothers remain appropriate. In France we still have the *Jouvence de l'abbé Souris, Contrecoup de l'abbé Perdrigeon,* and *Extrait de marron d'Inde* (extract of Indian chestnut). These three natural and inoffensive products, which "date back to the beginning of time", are none the less effective for all that, and are still available, thank God, in all French chemists.

A few minutes of daily gymnastics, skipping for example, and a few sessions of physical exercise two or three times a week (walking, jogging, bicycling, swimming) are particularly recommended.

One of the most effective exercises is never to take the lift but to go up the stairs slowly, two at a time.

– Fight against stress

Naturally, this does not mean trying to lower stress by taking tranquillisers or other kinds of antidepressants, but rather by doing relaxation techniques such as yoga or even sophrology.

Acupuncture, as well as some homeopathic or phytotherapies (plant healing), can also successfully contribute to the fight against stress.

– Use appropriate creams

The use of so-called "anti-cellulite" creams never meets with success if nothing else is done at the same time.

It has in fact been noted that when they are used in conjunction with the measures recommended above, they do help to obtain better results. Creams based on caffeine considerably improve superficial cellulite, but you must nevertheless avoid too deep massage which could "unstick" the nodules and make the cellulite which until then remained stationary "wander about".

– Miracle remedies

As far as I am concerned, there are two antidotes which may classed under this heading, even if some "spoilsports" will not fail to call them pure fantasies. The first of these is breast feeding.

Many of my previous female readers have told me that they lost their cellulite after breast feeding, whilst at the same time following the principles of the Method. This was not the case for their previous pregnancy.

The two factors together were therefore apparently necessary to gain a result: breast feeding and a change in eating habits.

Future mothers can always have a go! For the others, there is yet a second "miracle remedy", if you feel up to it. This is the cod liver oil remedy, which also has to be associated with a change in eating habits.

It has been effectively demonstrated scientifically that taking cod liver oil leads to a substantial reduction in fat mass, especially of the abdomen (see the works of Groscolas and Belzung).

Some people around me have tried this experiment by taking the daily equivalent of three soup spoons of cod liver oil for at least four months, whilst at the same time applying the principles of the Method. They have obtained interesting results as far as the diminution, or even the disappearance of their cellulite was concerned.

It is not difficult to believe in this, but it is difficult to try it, as it must be admitted that you need a bit of courage to undertake and carry on with the experiment!

For those who will stop at nothing, I would just say that the best technique for ingurgitating this "potion" is to put the lot into a glass (or yoghurt pot that you can throw away afterwards) and drink it down all in one go whilst holding on to your nose...You should then swallow the juice of two lemons, without sugar, of course. It is hard, but apparently it works!

– Drastic solutions

If everything we have so far proposed gives no satisfactory results, consulting a doctor specialised in æsthetic medicine is all that remains. The doctor will decide upon the most appropriate treatment according to the kind of cellulite. There are now many therapeutic possibilities: lymphatic draining, mesotherapy, cellulolipolysis, lipoject, lipo-endolosis or even liposuction.

The drawback to these treatments is of course, it goes without saying, their high price.

– Taking medicines

A whole chapter has been consecrated to this wide subject. Please refer to Chapter VII, Part II.

Water retention

We have already said that it is important to make a distinction between overweight linked to too much fat and that which can be put down to water retention.

Some women are in fact victims of oedemas predominantly of the joints, in the abdominal region and even their hands. These oedemas come and go, usually as a consequence of the menstrual cycle. Maximum water retention takes place before the period, and appears especially as in increase in breast and stomach size.

These symptoms are often accompanied by fatigue, loss of breath when making an effort, headaches, or even constipation, which may be linked to vein problems, anomalies in liquid distribution, and often too much oestrogen.

What can be done to limit its effects?

– You must begin by limiting salt consumption to a strict minimum, that is to say 5 to 8 g per day, avoiding everything that naturally contains it, such as pork products.
– Then, you should ensure that your food contains enough proteins by eating normal amounts of fish, meat, eggs and cheese.

– You must drink, as the best diuretic is water, especially Vittel water, and particularly as women suffering from water retention usually have a tendency to restrict their liquid intake.
It should be noted that water is even more effective as a diuretic when it is drunk lying down. This is a common practice in thermal cures.

– You should avoid taking any diuretic remedies, the effects of which are often open to question. They seem to work at first, but the body quickly adapts to them. When the treatment ceases the result is generally a worsening of the phenomenon.

– Should constipation occur, laxatives are also to be avoided. Only good eating will lead to a proper passage through the intestines (see Chapter V, Part II).
Circulation in the veins should however be treated appropriately. Treatments based on vitamin P (flavonoids) are particularly recommended.
Sleeping in a bed with the feet higher than the head, stopping smoking and lymphatic draining will complete the "kit" that will enable this unfortunately chronic affliction, to be treated.

How to stop smoking without getting fat

Statistics show an obvious correlation between stopping smoking and the risk of a large weight gain, which of course puts many women off trying to give up.

We now know why women smokers indulging in their little habit somewhat limit their weight gain.

Smoking effectively increases energy expenditure by stimulating the basic metabolism on the one hand, and speeding up transit through the intestines on the other, thus limiting the absorption of nutrients which are then eliminated in the faeces.

It would seem, in addition, that nicotine has the effect on inhibiting insulin secretion.

It is difficult to see how it could be possible to add the frustration inherent in a low calorie diet to the difficulties of giving up smoking [2].

Following the principles of the Method is the only way of doing this that will be not only acceptable but also effective.

And what if you're a vegetarian?

If following a vegetarian diet where you eat no meat is motivated by love of and respect for animals, this decision is commendable. If, on the other hand, this argument is based on the idea that meat is a source of "toxins" which are bad for the body, this is a reasoning founded on physiological arguments going back to the XIXth century, which have now been overridden.

These famous toxins do not mean a thing, as they are quite simply uric acid and urea, which are formed when

---

2. To find out more about this, see *Vivre sans tabac* (Living without tobacco), by Dr. Hervé Robert, Éditions Artulen.

meat is eaten. You should know that these substances are, in addition, perfectly well eliminated by the kidneys in a normal subject who drinks enough. The body is "programmed" to eliminate these metabolic wastes and manages it very well without any damage.

A vegetarian woman eating no meat, pork, poultry or fish, must however maintain a high enough intake of animal by-products so as to correctly balance her food. For this, she should try to eat milk products and eggs.

To meet protein needs properly, you need to have a good knowledge of nutrition and to know, for example, that animal proteins and vegetable proteins are not identical, and that some of them are only partially assimilated.

AMOUNT OF PROTEINS		
Soya beans..	35 g	100 %
Soya flour	45 g	100 %
Chick peas	78 g	70 %
Lentils	24 g	52 %
Broad beans	6.5 g	17 %
Whole wheat flour......................................	11.5 g	36 %

Thus, vegetable proteins do not have the same nutritional value as animal proteins and 10 g of proteins from lentils will not have anything like the same value as 10 g of protein from an egg.

This information is indispensable for those wishing to keep to a proper protein intake, which is 1 gram of protein a day per kilo of body weight.

Vegetarians who are also "great fans" of soya must also be aware that foods based on soya do not necessarily contain the same quantity of proteins.

Proteins contained in various products made with soya, per 100 g:

– Soya flour: 45 g
– Soya beans: 35 g

– Tofu (soya paste): 13 g
– Bean sprouts: 4 g
– Bamboo shoots: 1.5 g.

They should also be aware that soya juice, which is wrongly called "soya milk", is quite poor in calcium (42 mg/100 g) compared to cow's milk (120 mg/100 g); that vegetable proteins are lower in essential amino acids (those which the body does not know how to make itself), that the cereals are deficient in lysin, and the pulses in methionin. On this last aspect, I should point out that it is important to associate raw cereals, pulses and nuts (walnuts, hazelnuts, almonds, etc.) on a daily basis.

Additionally, many exotic old fashioned recipes systematically associated cereals and pulses:

– maize with red beans in Mexican tortillas,
– semolina and chick peas in Arab couscous,
– millet and peanuts in black Africa.

Eggs themselves, for their part, are very rich in, and have a perfect balance of amino acids.

A vegetarian has to be particularly careful about her iron intake (see above), because iron of vegetable origin is five times less well assimilated than iron of animal origin.

Also, to avoid vitamin B12 deficiency, they should equally try to eat cheese, eggs and seaweed.

Well-planned vegetarian menus are quite acceptable and can even be particularly beneficial to protect against cardiovascular disease and prevent some cancers (of the colon and rectum especially). They are, however, not advisable for small children (who are growing), and pregnant women and the elderly.

The Montignac Method is perfectly compatible with a vegetarian approach, as it advises you to eat a lot of carbohydrates (with a low glycaemic index):

- wholemeal bread
- brown rice
- wholemeal pasta
- lentils
- white and red beans
- peas and broad beans
- whole cereals and foods made from them
- fresh fruit and nuts
- soya and soya products
- high cacao content chocolate

The seven breakfasts of the week can therefore be based on bread which is rich in fibre or upon unsweetened cereals associated with a skimmed milk product, possibly flavoured with chocolate.

The Method also advises having a dinner based on good carbohydrates at least three times a week. Vegetarians could increase the number of this kind of meal.

The main dish could then be selected from among the following suggestions :

- brown rice with a tomato *coulis* [3];
- wholemeal pasta with a basilica, tomato or button mushroom sauce.
- lentils with onions;
- a mixture of red and white beans;
- peas or broad beans;
- chick peas;
- wholemeal semolina couscous without meat;
- soya based products;
- cereal based products (wheat cakes);
- seaweed.

This main dish could if necessary be livened up with a plate of vegetable soup, some *crudités*, vegetables, or a salad – finishing with a skimmed milk product (*0 % fat fromage blanc* or low-fat yoghurt).

---

3. See annexes.

It should be emphasised that a vegetarian diet which excludes all milk products and eggs and only relies on products of vegetable origin leads to deficiencies, and that means it is dangerous.

CHAPTER V

THE WOMAN OF FIFTY

A century ago, when a woman reached fifty, she stepped over the threshold of old age. The natural termination of her childbearing ability somehow rang the death knell of her "feminine" career. Between two hot flushes, it only remained for her to ply the art of being a grandmother.

Today, a woman of fifty is still a young woman and she has the means at her disposal to remain so as well.

Hormone replacement therapy (HRT), even if it is not really necessary, can effectively help her to pass through the menopause stage, or even to some extent prolong her youthfulness.

But, as always, it is thanks to the adoption of a way of eating that is nutritionally rich that she will be able not only to remain young, but above all foresee effective prevention of some health risks: osteoporosis, cardio-vascular illnesses, cancer, and also weight gain.

Once again, it will mean eating well to stay attractive, young and in good health, as one can be a grandmother whilst still keeping the body of a young woman.

The menopause

Menopause is fashionable. Or let us say that it is the time in the life of a woman which is particularly in the news. It is in fact talked about much more today than in the recent past, simply because the larger proportion of the female population is beginning to break the fifty barrier. This is in fact the slice of the population which corresponds to the post-war baby boom generation.

But the mentality of these modern women, who are the first to have known the pill, is different from that of their mothers.

The menopause, which was for the latter a symptom foreshadowing the beginning of the end, is only for their daughters an additional instalment in their feminine life. For, like pregnancy, these "liberated" women have understood that the menopause is not an illness, but just a normal physiological stage in their life as a woman.

Until the sixties, doctors were hardly interested at all in female sexuality and the feminine side their patients in general, except when they had to keep a check on pregnancy or child birth.

After the arrival of the pill, the situation evolved of its own accord. A dialogue with the doctor began on the subject of contraception, gynaecological problems and even sexuality.

As to the menopause, once rid of all its old symbols, it simply became the object of appropriate medicinal treatment.

1. What is the menopause?

It is the final end of reproductive functions and the hormonal secretion by the ovaries. The main outward manifestation of this is the end of periods.

270

The average age for the menopause is fifty, but it varies with race, climate and heredity. Though mothers and daughters often have their menopause at the same age, smoking will bring it forward by at least two years.

Modern woman, thanks to contraception, has managed to separate fertility and sexuality. This is why the sudden impossibility of having children does not upset her so much because she knows that her life as a woman can still continue.

2. The consequences of the menopause

The end of oestrogen secretion by the ovaries is the cause of many troubles which appear progressively:

- hot flushes;
- a more or less obvious urine incontinence;
- vaginal dryness with can make sex painful;
- dryer skin with premature ageing;
- beginning of osteoporosis;
- arterial lesions capable of giving rise to cardio-vascular illnesses;
- psychological and fitness problems which are a bit depressing;
- hormonal problems with sometimes an increase in weight.

Amongst these troubles, many can be prevented by the adoption of a particular kind of nutrition.

3. Eat well to keep young

Ageing of the human body is genetically programmed. But it may be speeded up by the aggressive effects of external factors such as free radicals.

Free radicals are toxic substances which are born in the cells in the course of chemical reactions in which oxygen is badly used.

The perturbations which they lead to have as a consequence the acceleration of cell ageing and reproduction (risk of cancer) and lead to vascular troubles.

A certain number of nutrients, which are classified as antioxidants, have the property of fighting against free radicals. These are:

– vitamin C,
– vitamin E,
– beta-carotene,
– selenium,
– zinc,
– polyphenols.

A well-adapted diet can help to give optimum amounts of nutrients.

NUTRIENTS	FOODS THAT ARE RICH IN THEM
Vitamin C	black currants, parsley, kiwis, broccoli, lemons, oranges, grapefruit, *crudités*, green salads.
Vitamin E	Wheat germ oil, maize oil, sunflower oil, walnut oil, grapeseed oil, wheat germ
Beta-carotene	Dandelions, water cress, cooked spinach, broccoli, lettuce, tomatoes. Dried apricots, mangoes, peaches, oranges. In fact, all coloured fruit and vegetables (orange, red or green)
Selenium	Fish, meat, offal, poultry, oysters, raw cereals, mushrooms.
Zinc	Oysters, dried peas, sesame seeds, brewer's yeast, liver, meat, hard cheeses, lentils, dried beans.
Polyphenols	Red wine, high cacao content chocolate (+ 70 %), tea.

4. How to protect your bones

Menopause constitutes the overwhelming factor for the onset of brittle bones. High calcium intake (preferably associated with vitamin D and hormone treatment) will be the best protection for your bone mass.

After fifty, the calcium ration for a woman should be from 1 200 to 1 500 mg a day. But, food studies on French women have shown that it is on average hardly 700 mg a day, which is insufficient.

As a consequence, after the menopause women should not only eat more cheese (especially Emmental) but should also avoid calcium losses which are accelerated by the absorption of alcohol (over half a litre of wine a day), coffee (more than four cups), and smoking.

It is also recommended that you have a bone mass assessment at the start of menopause (this is done with a scanner), which will enable the real risk of osteoporosis to be judged.

5. Hormone replacement treatment

Should the menopause be treated or not? The question goes far beyond the aim of this book and we would obviously have avoided it, if there were not weight implications in either case.

From fifty onwards, a woman in 1995 has a life expectancy of about thirty years. We may therefore seriously wonder if it is not wise to ensure her a quality of life which is necessary to achieve what still represents more than one third of her existence.

Keeping the skin more supple, so that wrinkles develop less quickly, preventing osteoporosis, the painful shrinking of the vertebræ which cause a humped back as well as hip fractures, these are the advantages that hormone treatment objectively leads us to hope for.

Added to this, absence of hormones makes someone who has gone through menopause more prone to cardio-vascular problems (inflammation of arteries, angina, coronary thrombosis).

There are certainly various (non-hormonal) treatments to alleviate hot flushes, but they do not protect the bones or arteries.

Only hormonal treatments with both oestrogens and natural progesterones are designed to prolong the biological balance which has been interrupted of its own accord by the years. Rather than an artifice this is, then, more in the way of giving a hand to nature, so that it can continue to do its work.

Menopause and weight

When they gain weight at the time of menopause, women are inclined to blame their hormones, the ones that have disappeared (if she not having HRT) or those that she has been prescribed.

Let's first examine the statistics, so as to have a more objective view:

It is obvious that we can note several facts when we examine these statistics:

Table I

WEIGHT GAIN AT THE TIME OF MENOPAUSE	
WITHOUT HORMONE REPLACEMENT	WITH HORMONE REPLACEMENT
52 % weight is unchanged 44 % gain weight (from 4-6 kilos) 4 % lose weight (from 2.5 to 7.5 kg)	67 % weight unchanged 31 % gain weight (4-7 kg) 2 % lose weight

Table II

WEIGHT GAIN AFTER HYSTERECTOMY	
PARTIAL HYSTERECTOMY *(removal of the uterus alone)*	COMPLETE HYSTERECTOMY *(removal of uterus and ovaries)*
35 % get fatter 56 % maintain their weight 9 % lose weight	50 % gain weight 33 % maintain their weight 17 % lose weight

Table III

VARIATION IN WEIGHT FOR WOMEN BETWEEN 52 AND 58 (OVERALL)
43 % are overweight (27 % of them are obese in the medical sense of the term) 52 % are of normal weight 5 % are underweight

Sources : Centre Européen de recherche et d'information sur le sur-poids (Dr. David Elia).

The statistics would not be complete without taking into account the general weight progression of women between twenty and fifty-two years old:

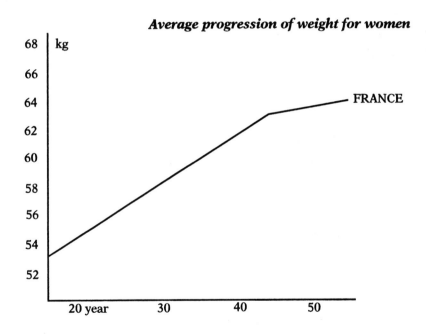

Average progression of weight for women

- Firstly, less than one women in two has a weight problem at the time of menopause (43 %);

- Secondly, weight gain is much lower when a women has HRT (31 % as against 44 %);

275

– Thirdly, it is highest where there is a total hysterectomy (50 %).

It is also important to note that the progression of average weight of French women is constant from adolescence, since for thirty years (between twenty and fifty years old) she gains about 10 kilos on average, going from fifty-three to sixty-three kilos.

Paradoxically, we even see that the progression in weight after fifty, that is to say at the time of menopause, slows down.

The experience of doctors leads us to observe, however, that women who put on weight at the time of the menopause (with or without HRT), are always those who are already a little overweight. Of these, 27 % are already obese, as shown in Table III.

It may then be concluded that, contrary to certain preconceived notions, menopause is not a determining factor in weight gain. It is only a factor which amplifies this for a subject who already is oversensitive to weight gain.

In other words, it is not the sudden absence of hormones, or even hormone treatment which is going to make women fatter, it is the metabolic changes induced by physiological transformation of their bodies which will lead to possible storage of reserve fats in a vulnerable person.

Well, how can we define which bodies are vulnerable to weight gain if not by measuring the propensity to hyperinsulinism?

It has been shown that lowering of oestrogens and even more so, their disappearance, had as a consequence the lowering of glucose tolerance and reduction of sensitivity to insulin, which quite obviously helps the onset of insulin resistance and therefore the increase of the insulin level.

The study by Wing, carried out in Pennsylvania in 1983, clearly shows the size of the phenomenon.

Level of insulin at menopause

EXCESS WEIGHT OF SUBJECT	ON EMPTY STOMACH	2 HOURS AFTER TAKING 75 G OF GLUCOSE	MULTIPLICATION COEFFICIENT
1 – 3.3 kg	48	260	5.4
3.4 – 6.5 kg	50	280	5.6
6.6 – 10.6 kg	52	320	6.1

This table clearly shows two phenomenons:

– first, insulinemia after taking glucose is disproportionate in the framework of the menopause;

– then, this disproportion is multiplied by the amount of excess weight.

In other words, the fatter one is, the more hyperinsulinism occurs, in the same way that the more hyperinsulinism you have, the more you will have a tendency to get fatter.

How to avoid getting fat during the menopause?

Both scenarios, with or without HRT, have to be examined separately.

1. Without HRT

This is the most awkward case, as we have seen that the probability of weight gain (from 4 to 7 kg) exists for 44 % of cases.

For those who are lucky enough to be slim already, or even thin, the risk of putting on weight is almost nil. If they have never been overweight (in spite of bad eating habits) it means that they have a cast iron pancreas and, consequently, it is hardly probable that this organ will suddenly start hyperinsulinism because of an oestrogen deficiency.

To be 100 % sure of this, all they have to do is follow the principles of the Method by going straight on to Phase II.

For those women who are already overweight, the problem will be much more difficult if they are a lot over weight.

The best solution would naturally have been to solve the problem once and for all well before reaching menopause, as we know that the latter does constitute a factor which leads to increased weight.

The fatter a woman is at the time of menopause, the more she runs the risk of getting fatter, and vice-versa.

Whatever the case, experience has shown that the application of the principles of the Method, especially following a very strict PHASE I, will give encouraging results and that it is in any event the best way of avoiding an extra weight gain. But you also have to take account of the other factors contributing to resistance to slimming, those that we enumerated in the previous chapters, just as you have to take into account the factors we are going to discuss at the end of this chapter.

Loss of weight by women of 50 and more when applying Phase I

BMI	AVERAGE LOSS OF WEIGHT AFTER 4 MONTHS	WEIGHT PERCENTAGE LOST
24 – 29	– 9.2kg	– 12.4 %
30 and +	– 15.1 kg	– 16.8 %

Source: Institut Vitalité et Nutrition.

2. With HRT

As the risk of gaining weight is obvious during menopause without HRT (we have seen that the lack of oestrogenes increases hyperinsulinism), you could be tempted to think that hormone treatment is the panacea.

Even though it presents incontestable advantages, it is far from guaranteeing that you do not put on weight, although this is statistically less likely than without the treatment (35 % as against 44 %).

Let us try together to understand why.

By their nature, oestrogenes can lead to:

– increase in the subcutaneous fat mass located on the femur;
– abdominal lipolysis;
– water retention;
– increase in the muscle mass (through the anabolic effect).

Progesterones, for their part, can lead to

– increased appetite;
– increase in the abdominal fat tissue (anabolic effect);
– water and sodium retention (mineral corticoid effect).

To sum up, an oestrogen/progesterone hormone replacement has the effect of triggering relative weight gain because of:

• possible increase in non-fat tissue (muscles);
• possible water retention
• possible increase in fat tissue.

But we now know that this possible and relative weight gain is conditioned by two parameters:

– possible prior excess weight and its volume (the fatter you are, the more risk of getting fat, and this is always because of hyperinsulinism);
– the choice of treatment made by the doctor.

As Doctor David Elias, gynaecologist wrote: *"There are no women who cannot support hormone therapy. There are only hormone therapies which are badly adapted to each individual woman. It must not be forgotten that an overdose or the opposite, insufficient amounts of oestrogens, is capable of provoking weight gain."*

There is therefore a "probation" period, avoiding under-prescription and over-prescription, during which the woman undergoing menopause will be able to maintain her weight.

Well conducted treatment does not lead (on average) to weight gain, on the contrary:

	BEFORE TREATMENT	AFTER TREATMENT
Average weight of women	57.1 ± 2.6 kg	56.8 ± 2.7 kg

This goes to show that the choice of hormones proposed, their strength and the precise adjustment of the dose are capital.

However, too often, doctors (and sometimes even some specialists) prescribe standardised treatments without taking into account the particular sensitivity of individual women.

It would be stupid to believe that there is a *"passe-partout"* hormone treatment for the menopause. There can only be treatments which are adapted or even personalised. Many are the practitioners who seem to care little about the æsthetic worries of their patients.

To exonerate them, it must be said that pharmaceutical laboratories do nothing to help them, as they hide the possible weight gain problems in general statistics which never differentiate between specific influences of hormones on women taking into account their size before treatment.

This is why a badly conducted treatment could make any woman put on weight, and particularly those who are already not slim. This means that HRT necessitates regular and attentive supervision, as the least weight gain should lead to modification of the dosage, or even question it entirely.

In the absence of precise explanations concerning mastering the risks of treatment, many women, because it worries them, do not try it.

This also why 30 % of women do not buy the medicines they are prescribed and 20 % give up before the year is out on their own judgement, even when they have started it.

That is why, even though it concerns nine million women in France, only 10 % of them are getting proper treatment.

To sum up, in the event that HRT for menopause is taking place, there are two measures to take to avoid weight gain:

1 – ensure that the treatment is adapted to your needs;
2 – follow the principles of the Method so as to avoid any additional risk of hyperinsulinism.

3. Slimming during the menopause

We have seen that the average weight gain for a woman between thirty and fifty was, according to the statistics, about 10 kilos.

Many women have so let themselves go, what with their badly managed pregnancies and the accumulated effects of bad eating habits, that they have, relatively, gained weight.

And it is at the time of the menopause, when they realise the risk of additional weight gain (with or without HRT) that they finally decide to take the bull by the horns and think of serious slimming.

It is never too late try, but you can imagine the frustration (not to mention the disappointments arising from lack of results in the long run) that the patient will endure if she has chosen to follow an "associated" low calorie diet like that of the good Dr. Jacques Fricker, or even like his cousin's, "Paul-Loup Sulitzer Diet".

Readjustment of eating habits, without any restrictions, such as the Montignac method proposes, is the only acceptable nutritional approach, and even more so since, as we are going to see, at the time of the menopause, women are often become a little depressed.

Other factors during menopause

The menopause may also provoke the advent of various health problems:

– thyroid insufficiency;
– depression;
– stress due to change of life-style;
– a more sedentary life.

In other words, the time of the menopause can give rise to various circumstances which could be indirect weight gain factors.

1. Watch out for depression!

The menopause is tiring. Once a possible hyperthyroid condition or iron deficiency are ruled out, the general practitioner should think of depressive circumstances which may be directly linked to menopause, or to things that happen around this time.

Professor A. Basdevant has examined the consequences of various psychological troubles on weight.

It can be seen, thanks to him, that their impact may go either way. You will get fatter or thinner according to your nature.

It can be seen that it is sexual difficulties that most often lead to a large increase in weight. They may even be paired with hiding a humiliating urinary incontinence.

TROUBLES	WEIGHT GAIN		WEIGHT LOSS	
	FREQUENCY	AMOUNT IN KILOS	FREQUENCY	AMOUNT IN KILOS
Depression	28 %	+ 7.8 ± 4.3	27 %	− 7.7 ± 3.6
Bereavement	9 %	+ 8.5 ± 4.3	26 %	− 6.7 ± 2.7
Divorce	15 %	+ 8.5 ± 4.3	36 %	− 8.3 ± 4.2
Family worries	14 %	+ 6.9 ± 3.1	14 %	− 6.6 ± 2.5
Marriage difficulties	12 %	+ 7.9 ± 3.1	12 %	− 8 ± 3.7
Sexual problems	15 %	+ 19.5 ± 25.3	12 %	− 7.8 ± 2.3
Financial problems	10 %	+ 7.1 ± 3.6	10 %	− 6.3 ± 2.5
Professional difficulties	14 %	+ 8.2 ± 4.5	8 %	− 6.5 ± 3.2
Moving house	2 %	+ 5 ± 0.9	7 %	− 5.6 ± 1.9

These weight gains give a good idea of how difficulties in having pleasure can easily lead to oral compensation through excess eating (generally bad carbohydrates).

Added to this, hormone insufficiencies linked to menopause lead to an over-reaction to stress.

Well, stress can favour secretion of cortisol by the surrenal glands. This has the following consequences:

- increase in abdominal fat;
- increased appetite;
- increased water retention;
- loss of lean tissue.

Hormone replacement therapy, when it is well applied, usually makes these difficulties disappear.

On the nutritional level, one should be careful to have sufficient magnesium, as this will help a woman to reduce her over-sensitivity to events around her.

2. Watch out for acidosis!

The problem of acidosis makes a lot of doctors laugh when it is brought up, as it is a condition that they do not often consider. However, it would seem that it is mentioned more and more often.

The number of anti-acid remedies available without prescription on the American market signifies a real problem. Dr. Catherine Kousmine for her part has given great importance to the good balance of basic acids.

Since her earliest publications, she has shown that modern processed food, too high in carbohydrates and meat, can lead to the development of acidosis. This, by stimulating a "sympathetic" reaction, leads to the following symptoms:

- fatigue, especially in the morning
- gastric acidity;
- bloating;
- constipation;
- coldness;
- glucose intolerance;
- psychological frailty combined with greater irritability and greater vulnerability to stress.

Dr. Kousmine therefore proposes limiting intake of acid forming foods (meat, strong cheeses, white bread, white pasta, sugar, alcohol, tea, coffee) in favour of alkaline foods (egg yoke, yoghurt, fresh fermented milk products, green vegetables, lemon, soya, fresh and dried fruit), or neutral foods (walnuts, whole cereals, wholemeal bread).

To control acidosis, you can also easily drink two freshly squeezed lemons every day when you get up, and during the day drink alkaline water (Vichy).

If you get acute acid indigestion, you can always fall back on the old remedy of bicarbonate of soda that our grandparents often used.

To check for yourself if you suffer acidosis, all you have to do is buy strips of litmus paper from the chemist and dip them in your second urine of the morning. The pH should be above 7.

Sport at fifty

Dietary convention based on low calorie theories will have us believe that excess weight is due not only to too high an energy intake, but also to insufficient physical exercise.

How then can we explain that Madame la Baronne, who never removes her stately backside from her Louis XV boudoir, and the bourgeois wife of a very rich industrialist who is unaware of the existence of a lift in her luxury apartment block in the 16th arrondissement of Paris, both conform to the ideal of being slim?

How can we explain that their chamber maids, cleaning ladies and other household employees, who are constantly physically active in their work, should be mostly "well covered", that is to say, weighted incontestably with excess fat?

Physical exercise and sport alone have never made anyone slim, and we have explained the technical reasons for this in Chapter VII, Part I.

This does not mean to say that physical activity is useless. On the contrary. But, once again, it is absolutely necessary to forget the erroneous concept of "energy expenditure" which is not significant, and to concentrate on the benefits to the body of normal stimulation of the muscle system.

Let us recall firstly that physical activity can only assist slimming to the extent to which (and this is imperative) you change your eating habits in the ways we have shown in this book.

After a first phase of weight loss, you can effectively help the system along a bit by taking up a physical activity. Exercising your muscles within the framework of the Method will enable you to:

– eventually increase glucose tolerance;
– lower hyperinsulinism, which will help lipolisis (therefore weight loss);
– reduce insulin resistance.

Physical exercise (in general) also improves the level of blood lipids (triglycerides, cholesterol, etc.), and lowers high blood pressure (if it was present), and this constitutes an excellent preventive measure for cardio-vascular diseases.

Let us not forget that, at the time of the menopause, a women loses the natural protection of her hormones, which makes her just as vulnerable as men to these diseases.

Physical exercise is also an excellent preventive measure against post-menopausal osteoporosis. But only regular and continuous training can be effective.

You could ask a physiotherapist or a sports doctor to draw you up a personalised training programme adapted to your needs.

Even if you do not have time, or the courage, to go in for an endurance sport, there are some basic measures that you can easily apply to your daily life. There again, all you have to do is change some bad habits and adopt better ones.

– Give up lifts and escalators. Take your time, but as a matter of principle, always go up the stairs.

– Walk as much as possible. If you live in a city, and you regularly take public transport, get off two stops sooner and walk the rest of the way. Walk at least half an hour a day. Go for a one or two hour walk at the week-end.

– Take advantage of your holidays to "budge", rather than lying on a sunbed. Walk along the beach paddling your feet. Go for outings on foot or on a bicycle in the country or in the mountains. Also do gymnastics and swimming.

Little by little, you will get to like it and what may have seemed boring at first will very quickly become a source of well-being. Gradually, as your fitness improves, you will feel more at one with your body.

Diabetic women

Diabetes is defined as the presence of too high a glucose level in the blood, both before and after meals. Two completely different types of diabetes can be distinguished.

1. Type II – or "fat diabetes"

This often concerns women around fifty and is usually accompanied by excess weight.

Technically we are dealing here with a pancreas which is secreting an excessive quantity of insulin. But as this hormone is "bad quality" or is not properly recognised by the body's cells, it remains of little use.

Hyperinsulinism therefore is added to insulin resistance. Glycaemia remains abnormally high as insulin secretion is not able to lower it.

Loss of weight is always necessary to enable glycaemia to return to normal. The principles of the Montignac Method are particularly well adapted to this kind of diabetes, because they rely, as you know, on the selection of low glycaemic index carbohydrates.

Studies have shown that a reduction of 14 % in the average glycaemic index of food (giving up white bread and potatoes in favour of wholemeal pastas and white beans) will improve the metabolic control of a diabetic.

A diabetic should therefore have food which is rich in fibres, and especially in soluble fibres (pectin in apples, alginates in seaweed, gums in white beans, etc.).

Their nourishment should also include quite a lot of micro-nutrients (chrome, vitamin B1) as these improve carbohydrate metabolism. These can be mainly found in raw cereals, brewer's yeast and wheat germ.

Diabetics should also limit and amount of saturated fats they eat (meat, pork products, butter, whole milk products)

287

in favour of poly-unsaturated, or better still mono-unsaturated fats, like virgin olive oil, which has properties which lower glycaemia and improve the balance of a diabetic.

The patient should not neglect to drink sufficient quantities (1.5 litres a day minimum).

2. Type I diabetes, or "thin diabetes"

This appears early, during infancy or adolescence. It is characterised by the fact that the pancreas is not functioning correctly and no longer makes insulin, which therefore leads to a necessary external input of insulin in the form of injections. There may be excess weight, but it is less frequent than in the first case.

Diabetics have a daily dose of carbohydrates to manage, which usually has to be spread over the three meals of the day. They should therefore try to eat fish and non-fatty poultry, associated with low glycaemic index carbohydrates (lentils, dried beans, brown rice, wholemeal pasta, etc.).

The richness in fibres of the foods we recommend for their nutrition can often help to reduce insulin doses, and in any case avoid hypoglycaemia.

For any diabetic, the risk comes from the appearance of cardio-vascular lesions (eye, liver and heart problems) which have to be avoided at any cost, so the preventive effect of following the Method will be particularly appreciated, though this should not be substituted for the advice given by your specialist. The Method enables you to be sure of:

– a choice of low glycaemic index carbohydrates which help lower bad cholesterol and triglycerides;
– contributing to increase in "good cholesterol" and reduction of triglycerides through a preference for poly and mono-unsaturated fatty acids;
– weight loss which often means that blood pressure returns to normal, reducing the work of the heart, making physical

exercise easier and bringing cardio-vascular risk factors back to normal;

– a diet rich in micro-nutrients (vitamin C, vitamin E, beta-carotene, zinc, selenium, polyphenols, etc.), protects the walls of the arteries.

This is how the nutritional options that we are recommending can contribute to preventing the vascular complications of diabetes, which are what make this condition so serious.

Female Constipation

Constipation is defined as "overdue" evacuation of faeces due to their dehydration. Constipation can be said to occur when the faeces are evacuated less than three times a week, as a normal person goes anything between three times a day to four times a week.

More than half the people in our society complain of constipation and amongst these, three quarters are women.

We can roughly distinguish two ordinary causes of constipation: either loss of the expulsion reflex, or slowed down progress of matter through the colon.

In the case of loss of the feeling of needing to go to the toilet, medicines, and often even a diet are ineffective. If the case is serious, therefore, a veritable retraining of the lost reflex should be undertaken, with, for example, the help of a physiotherapist trained in these techniques, which often call upon "biofeedback".

If on the other hand it is a case of lazy intestines, which it is more often than not, the treatment will associate:

– readjusting the diet;
– retraining the intestine, during which the habit of going

at regular intervals whether or not you feel the need will be re-introduced;
- physical exercise (walking, swimming, bicycle, gymnastics) to reinforce the abdominal muscles;
- an absolute stop to laxatives, as they are anti physiological. Over-use leads to a pathology of the intestines with hard to cure diarrhoea, stomach pains and big falls in potassium levels;
- giving up medicines that cause constipation, such as anti-depressants;
- stopping low calorie diets which cause a gastro-colon reflex;
- giving up some bad habits such as drinking paraffin oil, as they can be dangerous in the long run.

Feeding the constipated woman

You should start the day by taking a glass of fresh fruit juice when you wake up. This liquid, drunk on an empty stomach, will set off a gastro-colon reflex that will make you want to go to the toilet.

You should also enrich your food with fibres. Eating whole cereals (pasta, rice, wholemeal bread) and also pulses which are rich in insoluble fibres, should also largely meet the need. If necessary, you can also take 20 grams of wheat bran (from an organic source) mixed with a milk product (*fromage blanc*, yoghurt).

Sudden eating of large quantities of fibre can lead to bloating, gas, or even abdominal pain when intestines are upset and irritable. You have therefore to be careful to introduce them very progressively if this is the case. Begin with about five grams of bran a day, and increase it by five grams every week, until you reach the required amount.

Even if the intestines protest a little in the beginning, you should still persevere as these symptoms are benign and only a sign of encouragement to show that the colon is beginning to function normally again.

Your nutrition should in itself be able to bring you the desired amount of fibres, without having to fall back on various gums and laxatives which are sold at the chemists.

In addition, I would draw your attention to the fact that if you do not drink enough (less than 1.5 litres a day) this can make your faeces dry and difficult to pass.

To help empty the gall bladder and more effectively combat constipation, you can take a soup spoon of olive oil when you get up, and kill the taste by immediately afterwards drinking freshly squeezed lemon juice.

Finally, it may be said that treating constipation is even more important as it can indirectly prevent:

– acids from the stomach rising into the oesophagus;
– hiatus hernias;
– haemorrhoids;
– varicose veins which appear when the stomach is pressed as it often is by constipated people to try to get things moving.

Colitis problems in women

When we speak of "colitis" or of "irritable bowel syndrome", in every case, it is most often over-sensitivity to fermentation and food fibres in your large intestine.

This reacts by causing painful contractions or with an inflammation of its walls. Such reactions may be accompanied by constipation or diarrhoea.

When colon diverculosis is also present, a fibre rich diet is indispensable as it avoids infection and prevents this developing into cancer of the colon.

When there is clearly inflammation, a diet with no waste is temporarily necessary.

The following are then permissible:

– lean meat without any sauce;
– white rind and fat-free ham;
– lean fish cooked in foil or boiled in a little water;
– eggs cooked with no fat;
– gruyere cheese (or emmental, comté, beaufort);
– white rice;
– white pasta;
– semolina;
– sieved vegetable soup;
– cooked mixed vegetables: courgettes, green beans:
– vegetable mousse: broccoli, spinach, carrots, celery;
– peeled, cooked fruit;
– strained fruit juice;
– fruit jelly;
– butter, oils, margarine;
– non-effervescent mineral water;
– chicory as a drink.

However, this unbalanced diet must not be followed for too long.

If you only get normal colitis spasms (without diverticolisis), the problem is both simple and complicated. Because intestinal reaction is often painful, patients end up by gradually omitting an astonishing number of foods from their diet. Then you come to a point when restrictions are so drastic that nutritional input is completely unbalanced!

We see people who have given up everything made from milk, as they say that this is a principle cause. This serious decision may well lead to calcium or protein deficiency, and should not be lightly taken.

There are people who are allergic to the proteins of cow's milk, but this is rare and can be diagnosed by a complete check for any allergies by a specialist.

Lactose intolerance, lactose being the glucide (fat) in milk, is much more frequent, but it should not prevent consumption of fermented milk (yoghurt, cheese) which is always well tolerated.

As to foods which are rich in fibres, someone with a phobia about their colon affliction will tend to eliminate them altogether from their food. This is however a fundamental mistake as fibres will remedy the difficulties arising from passage through the intestines (diarrhoea or constipation).

But, for them to be well supported, you have to use them properly.

– You can start by calming the colon by going on a fibre free diet for a week, then re-introducing them very progressively, starting with tender green vegetables and peeled, cooked fruit.

– At the same time, increase your vitamin C by drinking strained fruit juices.

– Then, very progressively re-introduce raw foods: vegetables, salads, fruits.

– In the final stage you can add some bran if necessary, raising the amounts at a rate of 5 grams a week until you reach a dose of 20 grams. Eating whole foods can also be part of this programme.

– You have to remember to chew the starches well so that the enzymes in the saliva have time to work in your mouth, otherwise, in spite of the action of the pancreas, starch wastes will ferment in the colon and produce gases which are likely to cause discomfort.

– To alleviate pain or absorb the gas, you can take carbon or clay.

– If you suffer bad pains, you can resort to anti-spasm medicines.

– Finally, you must not forget that a rounded, bloated stomach is often the sign of stress. If this is the case, it would be better to eat in a quiet place, without hurry and with someone who you find relaxing. Meals eaten alone, that is to say with no convivial company, have a tendency to be eaten far too quickly.

– From time to time during the day, it is advisable to think of doing some breathing exercises, pulling in the stomach as far as possible. This will help to strengthen the muscle of the abdominal wall and works as a beneficial "massage" for the colon. Ten minutes relaxing after a meal can also be effective.

Apart from cases where there is really a personality problem, as when the faecal difficulty is upsetting the person's life, psychotherapy is not necessary. Lifestyle rules, nutrition advice and a good relationship with the doctor should be quite enough.

Nutritional prevention of cancer

In 1984, a conference organised on the subject of nutritional prevention of cancer, at the Anti-Cancer Centre in Villejuif (just outside Paris), seemed to the specialists present to be very incongruous at the time.

Today, things have changed a bit, to the extent that it is considered that 80 % of cancer comes partially from the environment and that food is directly responsible for nearly 40 % of it!

1. What is cancer?

Cancer is the result of the action of various parameters linked to the environment upon an organism with a predisposition, particularly in relation to the hereditary and metabolic criteria.

Under the influence of environmental factors, cancer causing substances come to play an "instigating" role, by entering into contact briefly at an early stage, with one or several cells in the body.

These cells are then transformed, so that they may potentially change and proliferate.

Then, a non-cancer causing agent, "the promoter" will enable the cells to multiply and eventually form a tumour.

The cell only becomes cancerous after a chain of abnormal sequences. Food is in fact only one link in the chain, but it may be determining.

2. Causes of cancer

The causes of cancer have been sought through various epidemiological studies. These took both geographical data and observations gathered on individuals.

Thus, in one case, the kinds of foods consumed in two different countries and the frequency of the same kind of cancer were compared. In another, the food consumption of subjects suffering from cancers was compared to people free of the disease.

But as La Vecchia says, *"studies founded on observation of populations are certainly useful to formulate hypotheses, but they can in no way bring us decisive proof of a relationship between cause and effect. A correlation does not necessarily imply links of causality".*

And as Professor Apfelbaum emphasised jokingly: *"It is not because France has the greatest number of Renault cars and holds the world record for cirrhosis of the liver that there is a relationship between these two facts!"*

Nevertheless, over the years, major directions for consideration have opened up. Even if their conclusions have to be interpreted with prudence, the work that has been done has enabled us to determine what foods and nutrients are likely to cause onset of cancer, as well as those which play a protective role.

3. Foods and nutrients which may cause cancer

a. Proteins

Cooking of animal proteins leads to the production of heteriocyclic amino acids which may be implicated in colon and rectum cancer.

This is why the risk for those who eat meat every day (beef, veal, pork or lamb) of getting these cancers is multiplied by 2.5 in relation to those who only eat it once a month.

On the other hand, protein deficiencies are just as bad, as they lead to immunity deficiencies through the slowing down of lymphocyte T activity, which enables cancer to develop more easily.

b. Lipids

Excess saturated fats in the diet seem to be a possible cause for appearance of breast, ovarian, uterus, colon and rectum cancer.

As long as Japan kept to its culinary traditions, which were poor in animal lipids, these kinds of cancer remained rare. But, with recent Westernisation of Japanese diets, breast cancer increased by 58 % between 1975 and 1985!

The excess fat in obese women increases the risk of breast cancer. Androidal obesity (apple shaped) is more dangerous in this respect than gynoidal obesity (pear shaped). Six times more breast cancers are found in the former, as accumulation of fat in the upper part of the body upsets the hormonal system more.

But you must not think for all that fats in general are the enemy to eradicate, as it is mostly the saturated fats in meat and milk products that are responsible. Fish, olive oil and evening primrose oil, for their part, may contain lipids with protective effects against cancer.

Any exaggeration is negative, and this is why you should not overdo lowering your cholesterol in relation to a normal level.

It has in fact been proved that a total cholesterol level below 1.80 g/l could lead to formation of a cancer of the rectum in the following ten years, which only goes to show that there should be moderation in everything. Particular care should be taken to see that there is always a proper ratio between the fatty acids, saturated and unsaturated, in your food.

c. Salt

Foods which are over-salted, including meat, pork and fish which have been preserved or marinated in salt can lead to stomach cancer. The Japanese are in a good position to know this, as they have paid a high price for their methods of preservation.

The frequency of stomach cancer has even so fallen by 64 % in Japan since refrigeration was adopted, and since they began to eat fresh products more frequently.

d. Alcohol

Alcohol is a cancer causing agent which works together with tobacco. However, its direct action is very badly understood as laboratory animals refuse alcoholic beverages. There is therefore no experimental model which enables a study to be made of the physiological changes it causes.

It is thought that one of the mechanisms by which it acts may be due to the fact that it seems to be a solvent, modifying the cells of the intestinal walls so that they allow cancer causing substances which are present in the intestines to pass through.

CONSUMPTION OF PUR ALCOHOL (IN GRAMS PER DAY)	RISK OF CANCER
30 to 40 g	× 2
40 to 80 g	× 4
80 to 100 g	× 10
more than 100 gr	× 20

France has the sad distinction of holding the world record for the number of alcohol induced cancers (pharynx, mouth, oesophagus, larynx, liver), and these cause about 14 000 deaths a year.

Let's remember that a litre of wine with 10° alcohol content contains 80 grams of alcohol. The association of alcohol and tobacco is even more poisonous. Thus, a litre of wine (or its equivalent in spirits, beer or aperitif), added to smoking twenty cigarettes a day, multiplies the risk of the appearance of cancer by fifty.

Do we need to remind you that one third of cancer is due to smoking which on its own is responsible for 90 % of cases of pulmonary, air passage, digestive tract, oesophagus and bladder cancers?

Oddly, even bad dental care, which is frequent in drinkers and smokers, increases the risks further.

People often complain that cancer is a terrible disease and medical research is going too slowly as it has not been able to find "the" cause and develop effective treatment. But let us reflect on this: the number of cancers would fall by 56 % if smoking and excess drinking were stopped.

e. Micro-nutrient deficiency

Beta-carotene, vitamin C, vitamin E and zinc are a protection against cancer, notably fighting the formation of free radicals.

Any deficiency in one of these micro-nutrients will therefore be a risk factor for cancer.

f. Pesticides

Professor Révillard noted that pesticides affect some liver and lung cells, which are particularly associated with immunity.

Among the pesticides currently in use, Carboryl inhibits the action of the white blood corpuscles and Lindane causes them to produce abnormal substances, which are similar to free radicals (adding to cancer risks) or like leucotrenes (chemical mediators which can cause inflammation, allergy and immune deficiencies).

g. Nitrates and nitrites

Water nitrates can be transformed into nitrites, then into cancer causing nitrosamins.   When you realise that in some French Departments, tap water contains up to 100 mg of nitrates, you can only be worried.

Nitrites were used for a long time in the preservation of pork.   You will not be surprised to learn that their use has fallen by 75 %, and that stomach cancer has also gone down by 66 %.

Some beers still contain nitrosamins, and are the cause of digestive cancer.

4. Cooking methods and cancer

Barbecues which smell of holidays and herbs can become flame throwers if they are not lit carefully and correctly, but the horizontal variety can be a time bomb.

When the heat melts the fats (lipids) in the meat or fish, it drips down onto the charcoal and on contact reacts and undergoes pyrolysis.   This phenomenon leads to the formation of cancer causing benzopyrene, without mentioning the other polycyclic hydrocarbons from smoke which impregnate the food.   This is why only a vertical barbecue is acceptable.

299

We have already mentioned that smoked foods (meat, pork, fish) were for a long time responsible for stomach cancer in the countries where such products were eaten throughout the year (around the Baltic and in Japan).

To this we may add that it would be preferable to avoid overheating butter, as above 130°C acrolein forms, and this is a substance that causes cancer.

5. Nutritional factors which protect against cancer

a. Antioxidants

Let us remind you of the list [1]:
- vitamin C,
- vitamin E,
- beta-carotene
- selenium,
- zinc
- polyphenols

b. Calcium

A calcium deficiency multiplies the risk of colon and rectum cancer by three. On the other hand, 1 250 mg of calcium a day for three months experimentally lowered the proliferation of tumour cells in the colon. This is why skimmed milk products are necessary, especially as they have had their saturated fatty acids removed.

c. Food fibres

We know that a lack of these can lead to lung, uterus and above all colon and rectum cancer. These are the insoluble fibres (cellulose, hemi-cellulose) which are the most effective.

Fibres have a protective action on the walls of the colon and rectum and this is due to several mechanisms:

---

1. Please refer to Chapter VI, Part I: table of vitamins.

– by decreasing the time that potentially cancerous agents (bile acids) are in contact with the mucous of the colon, and this is made possible by dilution of the content of the intestine (hydration of faeces) and acceleration of the time it takes to pass through:

– by reducing the time that the colon flora has to act on certain bile substances;

– by avoiding colon cell proliferation which the action of bile acids could cause.

It has been shown that greater intake of fibres alone does not have sufficient preventative action on colon and rectum cancer. It is also necessary to lower meat consumption for the protective effect of fibres to be real.

d. Unsaturated fats

Soya, maize, olive and sunflower oils (non oxidised) may have a protective effect against cancer.

e. Vegetables

Some vegetables contain substances which have been identified as protecting against cancer:

- indols in cabbage and broccoli, which de-activate oestrogen;

- sterols in cucumber;

- polyacetylenes in parsley, which block the early action of some prostaglandins;

- quinone in rosemary, which increases the activity of detoxifying enzymes

- isoflavones in many vegetables, which de-activate some enzymes which intervene in the genesis of cancer.

6. Some general principles to be respected

– *avoid over-eating and obesity.*
– *eat fish rather than meat, and avoid smoked and salted products.*
– *reduce intake of fats, especially saturated fats.*
– *add fibres to your diet (fruit, green vegetables, pulses, whole cereals).*
– *avoid vitamin destruction and loss of oligo-elements, especially during cooking.*
– *reduce alcohol consumption.*
– *try as often as possible to eat a balanced and varied diet.*

Even when cancer has been diagnosed, if is caught early enough (through heightened awareness), at the prevention stage and when the tumour can still be "controlled", all the mechanisms can still be reversed. There is, therefore, always time to change your eating habits.

Well conceived nutrition can represent an effective plus in minimising the side effects of possible chemotherapy or radiotherapy.

In addition to the nutritional advice, the general recommendations should also be followed. Cancer is not necessarily a fatality, and some cancer can even be quite simply avoided.

1. Do not smoke. Do not smoke on others.

2. Avoid long exposure to the sun (risk of skin cancer).

3. Respect the professional advice concerning handling of any cancerous substance.

4. Most cancers can be cured if diagnosed soon enough. See a doctor of you have any ongoing problems.

CHAPTER VI

THIRD AGE WOMAN: THE GOLDEN YEARS

The concept of old age is now completely old hat, but never has the popular adage been so true: *"you are only as old as your arteries"*.

In the XVIII century, one was old before one's age, to the extent that reaching forty was already an achievement and hardly 4 % of the population lived beyond sixty.

Nowadays, for the administration, we are "old" after sixty-five, whereas the life expectancy for a woman is now eighty-five. In 2001, more than 21 % of the French population will therefore be in the third age.

"Psychological" age, though, has little to do with chrono-logical age. Who does not know, amongst their acquaint-ances, at least one woman of seventy to seventy-five, if not older, who is still full of energy in spite of her age, and has no major handicap?

My own grandmother, who died prematurely and in good health at the age of one hundred and two, was a model of vitality.

On the day of her hundredth birthday, she even seemed much younger than most of the eighty-year olds who had come to congratulate her. Even though the psychological factor is important, it must be recognised that the eating habits of an elderly person can also be a determining element in their life span.

Even if the physical factors of ageing cannot be denied, the way in which a person eats is certainly the parameter upon which it is easiest to act in order to forestall the weight of age.

Natural ageing

Beyond an age situated around sixty to seventy, the body undergoes a certain number of natural changes.

1. Changes in body composition

Even though the weight of the organs and blood vessels does not change much, the lean tissue of the muscles does in fact diminish. This change can be due to lower secretion of androgens (and consequent lowering of protein anabolism), or to an excessively sedentary life-style.

All of this leads to decline in physical fitness and in turn to less mobility: ending with the risk of only going from "bed to armchair" and in the worst scenario, becoming bedridden.

Even though fat tissue increases proportionally in the abdominal region, sub-cutaneous fat has a tendency to diminish. As for the water content of the body, it is reduced in the following proportions:

– from 0.3 kilos a year between sixty and seventy;
– from 0.7 kilos a year after seventy.

This is why we commonly refer to an old person as being "wizened".

2. Functional changes

The digestive functions of an ageing body change as follows:

- alteration of taste, though atrophy of the taste buds, which is increased by a zinc deficiency. The distinction between salt and sweet is less pronounced. Food therefore seems more bland and this leads to the risk of overdoing sugar, salt and spices;

- dry mouth, due to an atrophy of the saliva glands, or the side effects of some medicines;

- reduction of chewing coefficient because of the state of teeth;

- increased frequency of gastro-duodenal reflux;

- slowing down of gastric evacuation;

- lowering of the secretion of pancreatic enzymes which makes it difficult to digest fats;

- lower level of digestive absorption, which increases micronutrient deficiencies: vitamins, mineral salts and oligo-elements;

- development of microbe proliferation which is a source of additional fermentation, because of slowing down in transit through the intestine.

3. Metabolic changes

These associate:

- slowing down of protein renewal by 30 % in relation to a younger adult;

- increased glycaemia after meals, because of insufficient insulin secretion, which it accompanied by an increased risk of insulin resistance;

– increase in loss of sodium and water which, when combined with lessening of thirst, accentuates the risk of dehydration. This can be identified simply be pinching the skin and seeing if the mark remains visible. This phenomenon is also increased by too frequent use of diuretics and laxatives.

Changes in lifestyle

Elderly people may be in one of two fundamentally different situations according to whether they stay in their homes or are "put away".

1. Women living in their own homes

Here again, two possibilities can be envisaged:

– those who do their own cooking or have it done by a member of their family or a household help. In this case their food stays normal and is unlikely to be too unbalanced;

– those who are reliant on food selected by a supplier delivering their meals to their home.

Many of these women, who are often widows, suffer from loneliness or isolation, and this results in latent depression which makes them anorexic and turned in on themselves. A vicious circle then occurs with the risk of gradual downward slide which, if it is not recognised soon enough can make the person become bedridden.

Excessive use of medicines is also often the cause of anorexia, digestive intolerance and sometimes even loss of micro-nutrients.

2. Women living in retirement homes, rest homes and institutions

– In rest homes elderly women have the benefit of cooked meals in a social atmosphere, as long as they do not cut themselves off by staying in their rooms.

– In institutions, or "long-stay" homes – we won't say geriatric wards – their food is supervised by dieteticians.

But, in practise, the situation is far from ideal, as elderly people only usually eat what they like! Food arrives cold or gets cold too quickly and there is usually not enough staff to help those who cannot do things for themselves. To blacken the picture even further, let us say that no-one checks on whether these elderly people have or have not eaten the food they were given.

Paradoxically then, it is in institutions, where the food is "measured" the most and where people are under the greatest supervision, that we see the more clear deficiencies and where severe malnutrition even occurs.

Deficiency malnutrition

Repeated nutritional mistakes can progressively lead to malnutrition inducing consequent chain reactions:

– fatigue leading to apathy,
– muscular wasting,
– loss of weight of up to 15 %,
– risk of falls and fractures,
– mental confusion,
– vulnerability to infections,
– intellectual deterioration.

Added to this, isolation and introversion, ignorance of some nutritional principles, impoverishment or even alcoholism, can only intensify the situation.

307

Preconceived ideas to combat

– An elderly person has high nutritional needs and must eat as much as an adolescent, especially as their intestine does not absorb food so well and protein synthesis is less efficient.

The food ration must absolutely not be lowered on the pretext that a person is elderly, less active and has less needs than others.

Any food restrictions of a low-calorie nature will create a source of micro-nutrient deficiency.

– An elderly person needs protein and iron. There is therefore no reason to ration them, by cutting out meat for example.

– You must not believe either, as some stupidly imply, that eggs are bad for the liver or that yoghurt leads to decalcification. These two foods must, on the contrary, be part of the nutritional selection of any elderly person.

In the same way, it is wrong to say that salt hardens the arteries, meat causes urea or that pulses cause bloating.

Eat well to live well

There is no "retirement" for food, this is why there is no reason to reduce energy inputs when a person reaches the third age. On the contrary, they should eat as they did before, continuing to have four meals a day, and neither the importance of breakfast nor the joy of English tea time should be neglected.

In 1983, Professor Le Cerf in Lille did a study which showed that the average calorie input of an elderly woman was 1680 calories, and her protein input remained often too low and unbalanced as more than 77 % of proteins consumed were of animal origin.

They should therefore think of eating whole foods, like cereals and pulses, which are also very rich in fibres and micro-nutrients.

Any protein restriction can only be made upon medical advice which will be given, for example, when there is severe renal malfunction.

If there are financial difficulties, they should think of eating eggs and milk which constitute a cheap source of proteins.

Making sure that they have a sufficient and varied intake of lipids should also be one of their concerns. In fact, as some enzymes stop working after a certain age, some fatty acids, which are no longer made by the body from the fatty acids in oil or butter, have necessarily to come from regularly eating meat, liver, eggs and above all, fish.

A good selection of carbohydrates is also a rule. In this regard, it would be best to always choose carbohydrates with a low glycaemic index because they are rich in vegetable proteins, fibres (which help fight constipation) and micro-nutrients.

On the other hand, you must not be too strict (except in the case of major obesity or badly balanced diabetes) about having a few sweet things which obviously are always a pleasure. Under this heading chocolate with more than 70 % cacao should be the first choice.

Be careful to drink enough and this advice is good for the rest of your life. Elderly people often do not feel thirsty, and adding this to the risk of functional dehydration implies the need for high liquid intake (at least 1.5 litres of water a day).

Soups, infusions, teas and fruit juice will be welcome. But excess coffee must be avoided as this leads to sleeping difficulties.

Get into the habit of drinking one or two glasses of red wine a day and at every meal, which is not only admissible but advisable, as everyone knows, wine has anti-oxidant properties and makes you feel good.

Calcium input for an elderly woman must be 1 200 to 1 500 mg/day and this is very important. But this is often much lower, especially when there is a restricted diet. Statistics show that:

- 58 % of elderly women absorb less than 800 mg of calcium a day;
- 16 % absorb less than 800 to 100 mg a day;
- 10 % more than 100 mg per day;
- only 16 % have a correct intake.

This deficiency is even more serious as calcium input of less than 100 mg is not sufficient to effectively counter osteoporosis (see Chapter V, part II).

Osteoporosis in elderly women is a little different from that which effects women at menopause, although it still affects vertebræ, which can shrink, but it primarily affects the long bones, causing spontaneous fractures as a result of small bangs, or falls. The hip and wrist are most often involved. This is why milk products are so important in feeding an elderly woman.

Vitamin D is also indispensable to fix the calcium. As it is made in the skin, upon exposure to sunlight, the importance of a minimum of sunshine for people in the third age will be recognised.

If they cannot stretch out in the sun as much as they would like, they can get this vitamin D from their food. To do this, they will have to eat about 12mcg (millionth of a gram) a day.

Foods rich in vitamin D

– cod liver oil	250 to 700 mcg/100 g
– tuna	60 mcg/100 g
– sardines	25 mcg/100 g
– chicken skin	20 mcg/100 g
– margarine	8 mcg/100 g
– egg yolk	5 mcg/100 g
– mushrooms	8 mcg/100 g
– pork	3 mcg/100 g
– chicken	2 mcg/100 g

Evident vitamin D deficiencies can lead to osteomalacia, which appears as pains in the pelvis and walking difficulties (it is the equivalent of rickets in children).

The general practitioner should always think of this diagnosis when he is faced with an elderly person having difficulty getting about. Vitamin D should then be prescribed in high doses.

Vitamin B9 or folic acid deficiency is also very frequent in the elderly. It is found in about 30 % of those living at home and 70 % of those living in institutions.

These deficiencies cause anaemia, but also, and more often, psychological problems: changes of mood, insomnia, wakefulness, depressive syndromes, apathy, and sometimes even senile behaviour.

It would be preferable to check this for every elderly woman who is "off her head" before attributing it to real senility.

A blood test, which is easy to do, could confirm this diagnosis. The remedy for this will be injections, but at the same time veritable preventive nutrition should be undertaken.

The daily ration of folic acid is 300 mcg.

Foods rich in folic acid

– brewer's yeast	4 000 mcg/100 g
– calf's liver	260 mcg/100 g
– oysters	240 mcg/100 g
– water cress, chicory	220 mcg/100 g
– cooked spinach	160 mcg/100 g
– avocados	150 mcg/100 g
– cooked red beans	130 mcg/100 g

Fill up on vitamin B6

We know that this vitamin helps to fix proteins for cellular renewal.

A vitamin B6 deficiency leads to fatigue, depression, abnormal irritability and greater vulnerability to infections.

Please refer to Chapter VI, Part I, if you wish to know which foods are rich in vitamin B6.

Do not go short of vitamin A

It is this vitamin that helps night vision and maintains skin and mucous in good condition. Daily dose should be 800 mcg.

Vitamin A deficiency (45 % of women over sixty suffer from this) will be responsible for dry and rough skin, greater vulnerability to pulmonary and ear, nose and throat infections, and abnormal sensitivity to sun.

Also give thought to:

– Antioxidants, and especially vitamins E and C as well as polyphenols, which actually have of the property of fighting ageing due to free radicals;
– iron;
– magnesium;
– potassium.

All the statistics show that the daily food of more than half of elderly people is very deficient in nutrient intake in relation to that recommended.

Be careful of diets!

All restrictive diets (low calorie, without salt, without fats, etc.) are dangerous for elderly people as they are the source of imbalances.

Some nutritional precautions can, however, be helpful in some circumstances:

– severe renal failure;
– serious high blood pressure;
– deteriorating heart conditions;
– very unbalanced diabetes.

As far as slimming is concerned, there are only two cases where a loss of weight can be medically justified:

1 – If the excess weight is a handicap to the person limiting their movement and they run the risk of being stuck in an armchair or in their bed because of their obesity, or if it is causing serious loss of breath with respiratory or cardiac difficulties;

2 – If an orthopaedic operation is anticipated for a hip or knee replacement. Apart from these two cases, it is useless, or I might even say, cruel, to force them to slim on a low calorie diet.

If the elderly person herself requests it, the general principles of the Method may be followed (PHASE II) as they meet the optimal dietary requirements. These principles should however be adopted in line with the previous observations, especially concerning nutrient needs.

Eating is for fun and meeting people

No diet will be balanced for long if it is not varied and does not respect individual tastes and preferences.

This is why the accent should be put on quality and presentation. Meals should be made "more gastronomic" to whet the appetite.

But it is the ambience, the environment and the happy social context in which an elderly person lives which will play the greatest role in the way they feed themselves. No-

313

one can disregard the fact that eating in the company of others always makes you eat better.

You have to try then to rediscover the hedonistic and Epicurean aspects of food, as this is primordial.

As Brillat-Savarin said: *"The pleasure of the table is for every age, all social conditions, in every country and every day; it can be added to all the other pleasures and is the last to remain and consoles us for their loss."*

Let us learn then to do justice to good food, and not be like Diafoirus [1].

---

1. Translator's note: Diafoirus: father and son in "Le Malade Imaginaire" of Molière, both ignorant and pretentious doctors.

CHAPTER VII

BAD MEDICATION

Some people are glad that scientific progress nowadays has enabled effective and appropriate remedies to be discovered for our illnesses.

But instead of using them in moderation and limiting their use to what is strictly necessary, in our society medicines have become widely used consumer products.

It has to be said that commercial pressure exercised by the flourishing pharmaceutical industry and its intermediaries has been such in the last few decades that systematic call upon medicines, even for the most simple ailments, has not only become habitual but a consumer reflex.

Doctors also greatly contributed to this "hyper-medicalisation" when they saw that their popularity was proportional to the size of their prescriptions.

If we add to this excessive use of prescription medicines the remedies that people prescribe for themselves, we get an idea of the size of the phenomenon, which would not be so bad if it did not have the unfortunate consequences on the budget of the health services that we have seen.

Unfortunately, this hyper-medicalisation paradoxically has health consequences. Medicines are not always, in fact, the inoffensive products that we think.

Their use, especially when it is excessive and continuous, can have serious perverse effects.

Side effects of some of them, including weight gain, are particularly noticeable. And those are just the medicines that women use the most.

Psychotropic medicines

These medicines are intended for the treatment of various nervous disorders. They act on certain centres of the brain (hypothalamus), which contain the "hunger mechanism" as well as the areas which regulate weight balance.

Hypophysis which regulates most hormone secretions of the endocrinal glands of the body (pancreas, surrenal, ovaries) also depends upon them.

Several kinds of medicines can be identified in the psychotropic family.

1. Antidepressants

Some of these, which are prescribed for severe nervous breakdowns, increase appetite and a taste for sweets, which can cause the complication of bouts of bulimia and eating between meals.

This aggravates insulin resistance as well (see Chapter IV, Part I).

If an antidepressant is really necessary, it would be better to prescribe one of the new treatments, such as Prozac, which do not carry risks of weight gain when there are no prior eating behavioural problems.

2. Neuroleptics

Amongst these we can name Largactil, Melleril, Moditen and Surmontil.

Like the ones mentioned above, they increase feelings of hunger and lead to a predilection for bad carbohydrates (sweet things particularly).

3. Tranquillisers and anxiolytics

Women too often have a tendency to fall for the "salvation" of the tranquilliser trap when they are going through a period of anxiety and suffering existential difficulties. It must be said that doctors, for their part, do not hesitate to prescribe them without difficulty as soon as they are requested.

This is how regrettable dependencies have arisen in countries where, even though they are not amongst the most unhappy on the planet, their inhabitants are however great amateurs of taking the famous "little happiness pills"!

What you may not know is that benzodiazepines (Lexotan, Lorazepam, Tranxene, Valium and Xanax) sometimes lead to problems of concentration and memory lapses which deprive women of the full use of their faculties.

These medications can, in addition, increase sensations of hunger and provoke a craving for sweet things.

4. Lithium

When this is taken, in the form of Priadel or Camcolit it causes intense thirst for sweet drinks. It also sometimes upsets the thyroid gland, thus creating another weight gain factor.

Given these observations, you should be wary of medicines which act on the psyche. Possible weight gain varies from one person to another, but could be from two to thirty kilos. In addition to increasing the risk of the appearance of illnesses linked to obesity, this kind of weight gain is

"Narcissistically" unacceptable for patients already suffering from a self-image problem.

Onset of obesity, in fact, often increases the psychological problems and then the patient will not stick to the treatment. When treatment is suddenly withdrawn because of weight gain, this could have dramatic effects and de-stabilise the individual to the point, sometimes, of leading them to commit suicide.

The duty of the doctor is therefore to weigh the necessity of the treatment against the problems linked to its side effects.

In some cases, the psychiatric condition may justify pursuing the treatment at the price of weight gain.

In a simple case of nerves, badly managed stress or negative thinking that will pass, you should be able to do without them, as it is possible to find the desired nervous relaxation by having recourse to other techniques. Women should especially try active therapies such as relaxation, sophrology and yoga.

Beta blockers

These medicines are prescribed to treat high blood pressure and prevent heart attacks due to heart weakness. However, their use has sometimes been extended to include migraine and some kinds of trembling, i.e. stage-fright for example (Inderal).

They usually cause weight gain because they reduce thermogenesis by causing a fall in sympathic tone.

They can, however, be replaced, with the agreement of the cardiologist, if there are cardio-vascular problems, by other medication with no side effects on weight (conversion enzyme inhibitors).

Cortisone

Cortisone causes weight gain through water and salt retention. It also upsets carbohydrate metabolism. This is why doctors rarely prescribe it lightly.

Its use is often justified during the development of serious illnesses where the prognostics for life or various functions is at stake (inflammatory rheumatism, allergies or serious infections, cancer).

The problem of excess weight is then of secondary importance and can be countered, when the cortisone doses are high and the treatment is of long duration, by adopting a strict diet free of salt, with controlled carbohydrate content.

Anti-inflammatory medicines

Phenylbutazone is no longer authorised to treat normal inflammation. But some treatments in the same category can, for some particularly sensitive patients, lead to a weight gain of two or three kilos.

Quite often, this is due more to water retention than to fat accumulation.

Here again, care must be taken before prescribing anti-inflammatory medication as it is not always necessary for just any kind of angina or dental infection, nor for rheumatism and period pains, especially as these medications can provoke digestive haemorrhages.

319

Antibiotics

Antibiotics are widely used for industrial farming as they enable a weight gain in animals of more than ten per cent to be achieved.

As the same cause will lead to the same effects, there is no reason why a mammal higher on the evolutionary scale such as man should escape the same consequences.

This is why antibiotic treatment must be justified and short-term. Long-standing prescriptions should only be used in exceptional cases and should be given with good reason.

It would be better to count on other ways of stimulating immunity and preventing the appearance of infections.

Tonics

As we saw in the first part of this book, fatigue is only a symptom. Tackling it by begging the doctor for a tonic is only a passive attitude which comes down to trying to treat the consequences of a result without taking its causes into consideration.

High doses of tonics have the effect of stimulating the appetite, and indirectly, causing weight gain. Some of them even contain amounts of sugar which are not negligible (vials, syrups).

Prescribing them, especially to children, can be a way of clearing the way to obesity.

Female hormones

We have spoken at length in previous chapters about the possible effects of the pill as well as oestrogens and progesterones during the menopause.

Other forms of medication can also interfere with nutrition, either by causing loss of taste (no less than forty remedies can do this), or by overworking the liver, which could then cause anomalies during food digestion.

Let us reiterate that good sense is always the rule. Some medicines must not be systematically prescribed for minor conditions, but only when they are strictly necessary, if they can be replaced by others which do not cause weight gain.

The doctor should then not only warn the patient of the risk of weight gain, but also take the necessary precautions to limit as far as possible the advent of possible obesity.

All this comes back once again to insisting on the necessity of a frank discussion between the doctor and the patient. The practitioner must know how to explain his prescription without at the same time painting too black a picture about possible weight gain.

We know that it is effectively difficult to evaluate this risk, taking into account the extremely variable reactions that can occur according to individual sensitivity.

Books written by Michel Montignac and translated into English, which are now on sale in the United Kingdom.

Dine Out and Lose Weight - ISBN 290623634-9   224 pp - **RRP £.12.95**

Michel's first book, originally released in France in 1986 and intended for the busy executive with an active weight problem. The English version has been revised recently, to make it more comprehensive and easier to read. For medics and nutritionists, there is an extended technical appendix at the end. A quality production, attractively presented, it remains a particularly suitable gift for the busy professional.

Eat Yourself Slim...and Stay Slim! - ISBN 291273700-1   240 pp - **RRP £.12.00**

This new title builds on the success of *Eat Yourself Slim* (first published in 1989) and brings the Montignac Method completely up to date.

The core message remains the same, but much new material has been added. Tables have been extended and greater attention has been given to the long term application of the Method - hence the amended title. In addition, readers are also introduced to a new concept called the Average Glycaemic Index, which replaces the "discrepancy management" of earlier books. This new concept is intended to help those embarking on Phase II widen their selection of food without straying too far beyond the bounds of good Montignac dietary practice.

Published in September 1998, *Eat Yourself Slim....and Stay Slim!* has become very popular with established and new Montignac followers alike, showing itself a worthy successor to the title it replaces.

The Miracle of Wine - ISBN 290623664-0   256 pp - **RRP £.15.00**

The title of this book us drawn from a chapter dealing with the health-giving properties of wine in his first book *Dine Out and Lose Weight,* Michel returns to a topic that still continues to fascinate. Written primarily for a French audience, its appeal and relevance is universal.

With 12 pages of colour, it is the ideal coffee-table book to complement *Dine Out and Lose Weight.*

Eat Well and Stay Young   ISBN 291273705-2   236 pp - **RRP £.12.00**

As we become more and more aware that eating good food matters, most of us still have little idea how to feed ourselves so that we can stay active into old age.

In this book, Michel Montignac shows us how.

Written originally for those entering their fifties, its message is relevant to young and old alike.

Recipes & Menus - ISBN 290623662-4   285 pp - **RRP £.15.00**

Still very popular, this is Michel's first cookbook, written to support those following the method. As its title suggests, the book also includes an eating plan based on the recipes.

Illustrated in colour.

Montignac Provençal Cookbook - ISBN 291273710-9   340 pp - **RRP £.20.00**

This all colour cookbook, redesigned and updated in 2002 in softback, firmly underlines Michel's gastronomic credentials. Designed to compete head-on with the best mainline cookery books, it has the added advantage of being entirely compatible with the dietary method and includes a three-month eating plan. Particular care has been given to ensure recipes are not only clear and concise, but also quick and easy to produce. A classic

The above title can be obtained from all good bookshops. In the event of difficulties, please contact our UK distributors

J H Haynes & Co. Sparkford

Order line: Telephone 01963 442080

                   Facsimile 01963 440001

                   sales@haynes-manuals.co.uk

VISIT
The Montignac Boutique & Café
Gourmet food store, Café and Wine Bar

160 Old Brompton Road
London SW5 0BA

Telephone/Fax 020 7370 2010
www.montignac.co.uk
mail@montignac.co.uk

For

Montignac wine and provisions, including bread.
Hot and cold drinks, snacks and meals all day.
Hot and cold food to take away.

A la Carte dining in the Wine Bar
Mondays to Saturdays – evenings only.

Store opening Hours
Mondays – Fridays 8.30am -9.00pm
Saturdays 8.30am – 6.00pm
Sundays 10.00am – 5.00pm

Mail Order
Via the above website, or call for catalogue

*Everything available in the boutique is
compatible with the Montignac Method*

USEFUL ADDRESSES

New-Diet
CUSTOMER HELPLINE
Michel Montignac Products
BP 250
92602 Asnières Cedex
Tél.: (00 331) 47 93 59 59
Fax: (00 331) 47 93 92 44

MONTIGNAC FOOD BOUTIQUES OPERATE IN

UNITED-KINGDOM

160 Old Brompton Road London SW5 OBA * °
Phone: 071 370 2010

FRANCE

1) 14, rue de Maubeuge
75009 Paris
Phone: (00 331) 49 95 93 42
2) 5, rue Benjamin Franklin
75116 Paris
Phone: (00 331) 45 27 35 73

---

* Mail order facility available.
° Catering.

THE FIRST NUTRITIONAL GASTRONOMIC RANGE

To permit those who have opted a healthy diet to find, on a daily basis, the main essentials of balanced nutrition. **Michel Montignac** has invented a range of exclusive products, specifically created using his own methods. These are all authentic products, rich in fibres and without any added sugar. All the products are aimed to bring to the body low-index glucids, a key point in the **Montignac** method.

Conceived by constant research on non-saturated fats and the absence of added sugars, this range is born of the rediscovery of the « all-included » the masterword of the **Montignac** method.

Indeed, all the nutrients that the organism needs are present in the wheat germ (vitamins, mineral salts, trace elements, essential fatty acids, vegetable proteins and fibres). The ultra-fine refinement of white flour strips the flour of practically all these nutrients, just leaving the starch. The « all-included » flour is a natural flour which not only conserves the totality of its natural caracteristics, but also assures a low-glucid index (35-40 against 70 to 85 for modern white flour) – depending on the degree of refinement.

This first gastronomic range is available under the **Michel Montignac** label in 400 shops in France and particularly:

– Numerous shops including the *Coffea* chain.

– Health food shops and particularly the *La Vie claire* and *Rayon Vert* chain of shops.

From 1995, a second range will also be available in supermarkets under the **Attitudes de Montignac** label.

To find out where these food products are available in the UK telephone the customer helpline (see useful addresses).

RECITES

COULIS DE TOMATES

Tomato Sauce

Ingredients

1 1b (500 g) tomato purée
3 large onions
2 garlic cloves
7 ounces (20 cl) basilica purée [1] (or equivalent in fresh basilica)
3.5 ounces (10 cl) garlic paste
3 soup spoons mixed herbs (Herbes de Provence)
1 yoghurt with 0 % fat content

Put the onions and garlic cloves through the mixer to make paste. Possibly add a little water to obtain a smoother mixture.

Put this mixture into a non-stick frying pan and let it evaporate on a very low setting until it has reduced to a purée.

Mix the tomato purée, the garlic and onion purée, the basilica, the garlic paste, herbs and yoghurt in a saucepan.

Cook this on a low setting for 30 minutes.

Note

This recipe contains no fats. It can therefore be used to accompany wholemeal pasta and brown rice.

See the book **"Montignac Recipes and MENUS"** if you would like to have a wider selection of recipes.

---

1. This can be obtained from the Montignac Boutique, 160 Old Bromptron Road, London, SW5 0BA, Tel/Fax 0171 370 2010.

SAUCE AUX CHAMPIGNONS
Mushroom Sauce

Ingredients

1/2 pound (250 g) tin of cèpe mushrooms
1/2 tin (250 g) of button mushrooms
7 ounces (20 cl) cream
3.5 ounces (5-6 cl) garlic paste
freeze-dried tarragon
salt and pepper

Drain the cèpe mushrooms then cut them into fine slices. Fry them lightly for a few minutes in a little olive oil.

Put the drained button mushrooms in the mixer, with half the cèpe mushrooms and make a purée. If necessary, moisten with a little of the cream.

In a saucepan, add the rest of the cèpe mushrooms to the mushroom purée, add the basilica purée, the garlic paste and the rest of the cream. Season with salt, pepper and tarragon.

Cook on very low setting to avoid sticking to the bottom of the saucepan.

Note

Cèpe mushrooms are not obligatory, and the recipe can be made up with 500 g of button mushrooms.

If you are making a **PHASE I** recipe, then the 20 cl of cream should be replaced with a 0 % fat yoghurt or the equivalent amount of *fromage blanc*.

Printed in Great Britain by J. H. Haynes & Co. Ltd.